Malena Johannes

Big Data for Big Pharma

An Accelerator for
The Research and Development Engine?

SCHRIFTENREIHE MASTERSTUDIENGANG CONSUMER HEALTH CARE

herausgegeben von Prof. Dr. Marion Schaefer

ISSN 1869-6627

13 *Dirk Klintworth*
Reporting Guidelines und ihre Bedeutung für die Präventions- und Gesundheitsförderungsforschung
ISBN 978-3-8382-0448-2

14 *Judith Weigel*
Schwangerschaft bei Frauen mit und ohne Autoimmunerkrankungen
Ein Vergleich hinsichtlich der mütterlichen Charakteristika und des Ausgangs der Schwangerschaft
ISBN 978-3-8382-0468-0

15 *Christopher Funk*
Mobile Softwareanwendungen (Apps) im Gesundheitsbereich
Entwicklung, Marktbetrachtung und Endverbrauchermeinung
ISBN 978-3-8382-0493-2

16 *Carmen Flecks*
Auf der Suche nach Psychotherapie
Bedarfsplanung für die Psychotherapie unter besonderer Berücksichtigung des Versorgungsstrukturgesetzes 2012 (GKV-VStG)
ISBN 978-3-8382-0498-7

17 *Beate Kern*
Arzneimittel für seltene Erkrankungen:
Evidenzlevel der Wirksamkeitsstudien, Frühe Nutzenbewertung und Preisentwicklung in Deutschland
ISBN 978-3-8382-0762-9

18 *Heike Dally*
Anforderungen an das Design klinischer Studien in der Onkologie nach Einführung der frühen Nutzenbewertung
ISBN 978-3-8382-0933-3

19 *Malena Johannes*
Big Data for Big Pharma
An Accelerator for The Research and Development Engine?
ISBN 978-3-8382-0942-5

Malena Johannes

BIG DATA FOR BIG PHARMA

AN ACCELERATOR FOR
THE RESEARCH AND DEVELOPMENT ENGINE?

ibidem-Verlag
Stuttgart

Bibliografische Information der Deutschen Nationalbibliothek
Die Deutsche Nationalbibliothek verzeichnet diese Publikation in der Deutschen Nationalbibliografie; detaillierte bibliografische Daten sind im Internet über http://dnb.d-nb.de abrufbar.

Bibliographic information published by the Deutsche Nationalbibliothek
Die Deutsche Nationalbibliothek lists this publication in the Deutsche Nationalbibliografie; detailed bibliographic data are available in the Internet at http://dnb.d-nb.de.

∞

Gedruckt auf alterungsbeständigem, säurefreien Papier
Printed on acid-free paper

ISBN-13: 978-3-8382-0942-5

© *ibidem*-Verlag
Stuttgart 2016

Alle Rechte vorbehalten

Das Werk einschließlich aller seiner Teile ist urheberrechtlich geschützt. Jede Verwertung außerhalb der engen Grenzen des Urheberrechtsgesetzes ist ohne Zustimmung des Verlages unzulässig und strafbar. Dies gilt insbesondere für Vervielfältigungen, Übersetzungen, Mikroverfilmungen und elektronische Speicherformen sowie die Einspeicherung und Verarbeitung in elektronischen Systemen.

All rights reserved. No part of this publication may be reproduced, stored in or introduced into a retrieval system, or transmitted, in any form, or by any means (electronical, mechanical, photocopying, recording or otherwise) without the prior written permission of the publisher. Any person who does any unauthorized act in relation to this publication may be liable to criminal prosecution and civil claims for damages.

Printed in Germany

Structure

List Of Figures 6

Abbreviations 7

Summary 9

1. Introduction 11
2. Objectives And Scope 13
3. The Innovation Gap In R&D For The Pharmaceutical Industry 15
   3.1 Challenges Of The Innovation Process 15
   3.2 Measures Big Pharma Is Taking To Address The Challenges 21
4. Can Big Data Overcome The Innovation Gap? 23
   4.1 Big Data: Definition 23
   4.2 Areas Of Use Within The Pharmaceutical Industry 26
   4.3 Key Hurdles For The Acquisition And Analysis Of Big Data 28
   4.4 Legal Implications 31
5. Online Research: Use And Impact Of Big Data For R&D Among Top 5 Pharmaceutical Companies 37
   5.1 Methodology 37
   5.2 Results 38
      5.2.1 Novartis 38
      5.2.2 Pfizer: 43
      5.2.3 Sanofi 49
      5.2.4 Roche 52
      5.2.5 Merck & Co 59
   5.3 Interpretation And Analysis 63
6. Conclusion: Derived Strategies To Leverage Big Data For R&D 71
   6.1 Infrastructure 72
   6.2 Interoperability 74
   6.3 Big Data Business Intelligence 75
7. Key Findings And Future Outlook 79
8. Reference List 81
9. Appendices 94

List of Figures

Figure 1: Top 5 Global Pharmaceutical Companies based on Pharma Revenue in 2014..13
Figure 2: The phases of clinical development, registration and launch & sales......15
Figure 3: The traditional R&D process and principle timelines of a new compound..16
Figure 4: Total R&D expenditures of PhRMA members from 1995-2012.........19
Figure 5: NMEs approved by FDA between 2001 and 2012 by major pharmaceutical companies..20
Figure 6: Volume and format of data created every minute online................24
Figure 7: The Characteristics of Big Data – The 3 Vs.................................25
Figure 8: The opportunities for Big Data within the product value chain...........28
Figure 9: Four distinct data pools and their owners..................................29
Figure 10: Required integration of data pools to unlock the full potential of Big Data...30
Figure 11: 'Spheres' of protection of healthcare information........................32
Figure 12: Big Data and privacy issues...35
Figure 13: Summary of the results of the online research..........................72
Figure 14: The 7 dimensions of data quality..73
Figure 15: The Big Data framework for pharmaceutical companies................75
Figure 16: Big Data management within an organization...........................76
Figure 17: Overview of key components of Big Data Governance.................77
Figure 18: The process of implementing Big Data in alignment with the overall corporate strategy..78

Abbreviations

EU	European Union
FDA	Food and Drug Administration
HTA	Health Technology Assessment
HDFS	The Hadoop Distributed File System
HQL	Hive Query Language
NGS	Next Generation Sequencing
NME	New Molecular Entity
NoSQL	Non-Relational Structure Query Language
PhRMA	The Pharmaceutical Research and Manufacturers of America
R&D	Research and Development
RWD	Real World Data
RWE	Real World Evidence
SQL	Structure Query Language

Summary
Large amounts of digital data, from geographic location to data search history, are generated automatically with any online activity. The increasing number of people, devices, and sensors connected by digital networks further expands this body of data. The ability to store trillions of bytes of information and the constant research into analytics tools to extract value from the unstructured data flood, collectively known as 'Big Data', has the potential to positively support businesses in many industry sectors including healthcare.

In the last two decades, the pharmaceutical industry has seen a steadily decline in research and development (R&D) productivity caused by increasing costs, while the number of new pharmaceutical compounds obtaining market authorization has been stagnant, driven by ever-increasing regulatory hurdles and mounting difficulty in finding the next blockbuster drug (either in a new disease area or a far superior product to what is currently in the market). The pharmaceutical industry has looked at many ways to address the innovation gap, starting with increased R&D spending, followed by major consolidations, in-licensing, acquisitions and R&D reorganization – but to no avail. Big Data experts claim that the pharmaceutical industry needs to take better advantage of today´s data phenomenon and look into ways to connect disparate data from external sources in the healthcare world in order to reinvigorate the R&D engine.

In fact, pharmaceutical companies have started to embrace Big Data for their R&D process, but the big question remains whether this hype will help to accelerate drug innovations. This study examines this question by conducting an online research looking at the top five pharmaceutical companies ('Big Pharma') by revenue in 2014 – Novartis, Pfizer, Sanofi, Roche and Merck & Co. The results demonstrate that all of the examined companies have started to implement Big Data for R&D, in particular in the field of oncology, to help identify and validate new drug targets and improve patient stratification. Though it is too early to draw definite conclusions of the impact that Big Data can have for the R&D engine, there are signs that Big Data can contribute to the successful completion of clinical trials. Big Pharma's utilization of Big Data is still in the early stages and the industry will need to continue investigating how to best implement and use Big Data for its business needs and research focus to extract the most value out of the data explosion.

1. Introduction

"We have discovered the cure for cancer, we just can't find it."[1]
(Research and Development Executive, Global Pharmaceutical Company)

Evolutions in technology, increasing digitalization, and an era of open information - there are many reasons that have led to the massive, hard-to-handle amounts of unstructured data. Big Data has become the buzzword of the decade. Industry leaders have started to embrace the data phenomenon and aim to unlock the claimed business potential. Ironically, the pharmaceutical industry is one of the industries that late joined the Big Data hype, although no other industry is and has always been more dependent on data. Any new drug that a pharmaceutical company brings to market has to demonstrate an extensive set of clinical trial data to prove a positive benefit-risk profile in order to seek marketing authorization. Furthermore, data determines any business decision within the research and development (R&D) process, the heart of the risky business a pharmaceutical company has to face. The development of a new drug is an investment of around US$2 billion and takes on average 14 years.[2] Any failure is a huge financial loss, and in fact, failures are not rare. Out of over 200 pipeline projects per company per year[3] (see appendix 1 for more details), only 0.6 new pharmaceutical compounds make it to the market[4]. The Big Data buzz claims to have the potential to reduce costs and time by improving patients' outcomes at the same time. Moreover, Big Data claims to open new ways of research pathways resulting in, for instance, personalized cancer drugs that would never have made it to the market a decade ago as clinical trials were not designed to meet niche patients' needs and as such, would not have met the targeted clinical endpoints.

Big Data claims to be full of insights that Big Pharma need to find a way of harvesting, which could lead to new compounds. Academics, Big Data start-ups and pharmaceutical companies have focused their research efforts on analytic tools and data technologies to store, collect, analyse and extract these insights from massive data sets. However, the key question is whether the Big Data hype really does have the claimed revolutionary effect on the complex R&D process or if it actually

---

[1] iNFORMATICA (2013), p.1
[2] Ding et al. (2014), p.4
[3] Citeline (2015), p.6
[4] Schuhmacher (2015), p. 45

creates another hurdle for Big Pharma innovation? The goal of this research is to shed light on this question.

2. Objectives and scope

The objective of this study is to examine whether and how the top 5 pharmaceutical companies are applying Big Data for their R&D processes as well as to whether Big Data initiatives have proven to increase R&D efficiency. Based on the pharma revenue in 2014, the latest figures show that Novartis, Pfizer, Sanofi, Roche and Merck & Co. are currently the five leading pharmaceutical companies and have thus been selected as the subjects of this research.

Figure 1: Top 5 Global Pharmaceutical Companies based on Pharma Revenue in 2014
Source: Statista (2015)

Thereby, the following key questions will be examined:
- Which of the top 5 global pharmaceutical companies are active in the field of Big Data and R&D?
- What are the areas within the innovation process of a new pharmaceutical compound that pharmaceutical companies are most interested to utilize Big Data to inform strategies?
- If the information is available: How much do Big Pharma invest into Big Data strategies for R&D from a financial and resourcing perspective?
- Have the selected pharmaceutical companies initiated collaborations with other pharmaceutical, biotech or IT companies/research institutes or other stakeholders within the healthcare sector concerning this matter?
- Is Big Pharma still in the experimental stage or are there already Best Practice Cases available on successful Big Data activities for R&D?
- Have Big Data initiatives proven to demonstrate a higher success rate for the overall R&D process than traditional R&D approaches?

3. The innovation gap in R&D for the pharmaceutical industry

3.1 Challenges of the innovation process

Innovation in the pharmaceutical sector is a highly complex, lengthy and risky process. No other industry is significantly more linked to science and more regulated.

The traditional innovation process is divided into preclinical research including drug discovery and preclinical testing, clinical development (phase I-III) and a regulatory review and finally, the launch phase.[5]

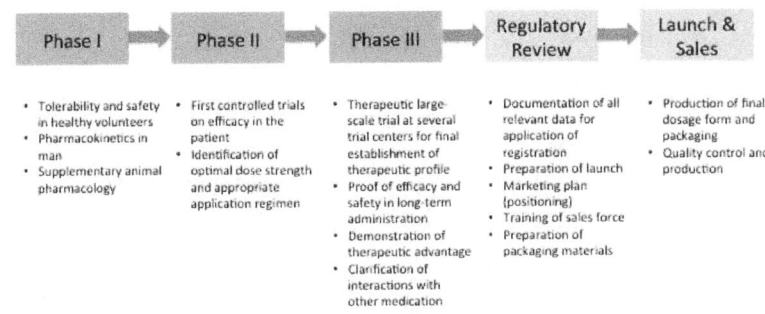

Figure 2: The phases of clinical development, registration and launch & sales
Source: Own illustration based on Gassmann (2015), p.64-65

While the process of developing and bringing one new compound to the market takes on average 14 years, another specific characteristic is that pharmaceutical R&D also faces a low probability of success. Only one of more than 100,000 compounds that have been screened in discovery research make it to the market – even from the discovery stage, the number is whittled down to one in 10 by the pre-clinical research phase. In fact, the probability of discovering, developing and registering a new molecular entity has been estimated to be only around 4%, which makes it a risky and cost-intense business.[6]

---

[5] Gassmann (2015), p.64-65
[6] Schuhmacher (2015), p.47

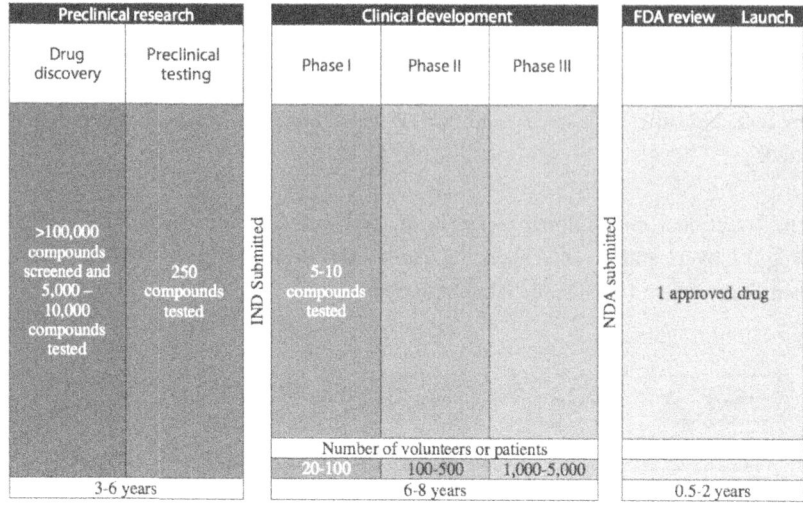

Figure 3: The traditional R&D process and principle timelines of a new compound
Source: Schuhmacher (2015), p.46

According to Ding et al. the complexity of the innovation process in the pharmaceutical industry can be described by the following three characteristics: *Live or die, large in size, and finite lifespan.*

Live or die is the pragmatic expression for the risky business that pharmaceutical companies have to face. A pharmaceutical company can only survive if its R&D efforts pay off. In other words, an empty pipeline, failures of drug compounds during the clinical phase resulting in the absence of drug launches puts a pharmaceutical company at risk.

Large in size refers to the fact that each new drug tends to generate a large amount of revenue for a firm. A successful so-called blockbuster product that generates at least US$ 1 billion per year in revenue can outweigh the costs for failed research; in turn, a firm´s loss of income from a drug compound is usually accompanied by a significant drop in the overall performance and profit. Hence, pharmaceutical companies face the ongoing challenge of delivering consistent results and ensuring stable and successful innovation.

Finite lifespan means the limited time that a new innovative drug will be valuable and bring in significant revenue to "pay back" the R&D costs. The standard lifespan of a drug is defined by the patent validity.[7] As soon as the drug´s patent expires, generics will enter the market and take over a high segment of market share, leading to a significantly revenue decrease of up to 90%.[8] To put numbers into perspective, projected revenues of all new molecular entities between 2012-2016 are expected to be US$58 billion whereas losses by patent expirations are forecasted to be US$123 billion.[9] In addition, it is worth noting that only 3 out of 10 drugs generate revenue that meet or exceed average R&D costs.[10]

Therefore, a pharmaceutical company has to consider and balance the following four key dimensions: cost, uncertainty, return and time.

Cost:

The costs for the development of a new drug are immense. Excluding any other factors and assuming the development for a drug takes 14 years, today´s total costs for R&D per compound is US$1.8 billion.[12] An increase in the interest rate and any prolongation of the R&D timeline has a negative impact on costs. Further, costs of R&D have risen rapidly over the last decades and have doubled every 8.5 years since 1950[12], driven by larger and more complex clinical studies and expensive new enabling technologies. Before 1990s, the R&D costs were less than US$250 million; in 2000, the costs rose to US$803 million and by 2005 surpassed the US $ 1 billion mark (approximately US$1.3 billion[11]). Since then, costs have steadily increased and are expected to soon hit US$2 billion. The clinical development phases, from Phase I to submission, account for 63% of these total R&D costs.[12] Consequently, the costs of developing a new compound have an impact on the innovation decision and hence limit the number of new drug projects that a firm can support at a given time.[13]

---

[7] Ding et al. (2014)
[8] European Commission (1) (2013), p.59
[9] Schuhmacher (2015), p.64
[10] Gassmann (2008), p. 1
[11] Petrova (2014), p.25
[12] Schuhmacher (2015), p. 52
[13] Ding et al. (2014), p.4

Uncertainty:
Uncertainty is related to the low rate of probability of success for a new molecular entity to come to the market. Each phase of the innovation process entails the risk that a drug can fail for various reasons. A review of the FDA in 2012 demonstrated that most failures at Phase II and Phase III resulted from insufficient efficacy of the drug demonstrated (56%), followed by safety concerns (28%). Differences in attrition rates may depend on the drug class, the therapeutic area, the type of disease, the source of the drug candidate (self-originated drugs vs. in-licensed drugs), and the size of the company. For example, central nervous system (CNS) drug candidates have a higher probability of failure in later stage clinical trials due to the lack of predictive animal models in the discovery research and the pre-clinical testing phase.[14]

Return (of investment):
Return of investment is closely associated with uncertainty. Key for sustainability is the balance of uncertainty with potential return. As mentioned before, each new drug has the potential to create substantial value for the company. As such, a pharmaceutical company must select innovation projects that can potentially provide large-scale return to at least make up for future lost income due to patent expirations of existing blockbuster drug or failures during the R&D process. In turn and conditional upon this, the executive board of a pharmaceutical company must also assess how much uncertainty it is willing to bear to target an even larger return. First-in-class innovations result in higher revenue, but have higher attrition rates. Me-too drugs[15] have a lower potential of large-scale revenue, but the development process is less risky and the probability rate of success is significantly higher.

Time:
Time is not only measured as how long it takes to develop and bring a drug to market, but also includes the limited length of patent protection of a new molecular entity. The majority of the income of a pharmaceutical company comes from drugs with patent protection so it is critical for a firm to plan ahead and initiate new clinical trial programmes to ensure new drug compounds are available for

---

[14] Schuhmacher (2015), p.47
[15] Drugs that are structurally very similar to already known drugs, with only minor differences.

launch when patents of existing blockbusters expire to replace the expected loss of revenue.

A number of mega trends have arisen in the last decade that also have challenged the pharmaceutical R&D process:

- *Decline of R&D efficiency*
  The pharmaceutical industry has seen a steadily decline of R&D efficiency since 1950 and this is expected to be continued given the challenging landscape. This is because while the number of new drugs launched by the industry has been constant, the costs per new drug have continuously increased (see table below) due to the following reasons:
    o New technologies in drug research, such as combinatorial chemistry, DNA sequencing, high throughput screening, and computational drug design
    o The increasing size of clinical trials
    o The increasing costs for clinical infrastructure
    o A greater complexity of clinical trials conducted for drugs to treat chronic diseases
    o A higher number of R&D personnel[16]

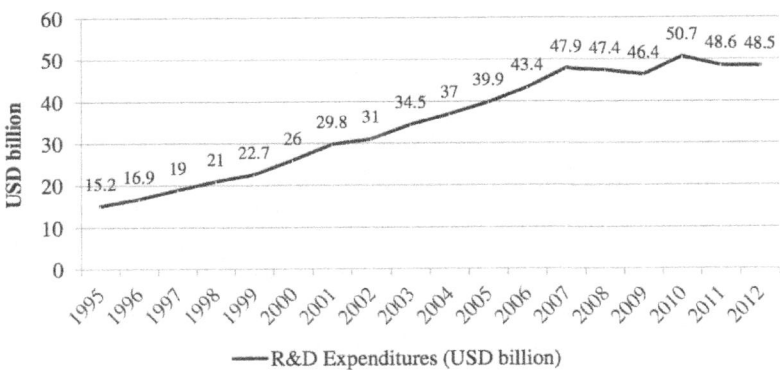

Figure 4: Total R&D expenditures of PhRMA[17] members from 1995-2012
Source: Schuhmacher (2015), p.58

---

[16] Schuhmacher (2015), p.52
[17] The Pharmaceutical Research and Manufacturers of America

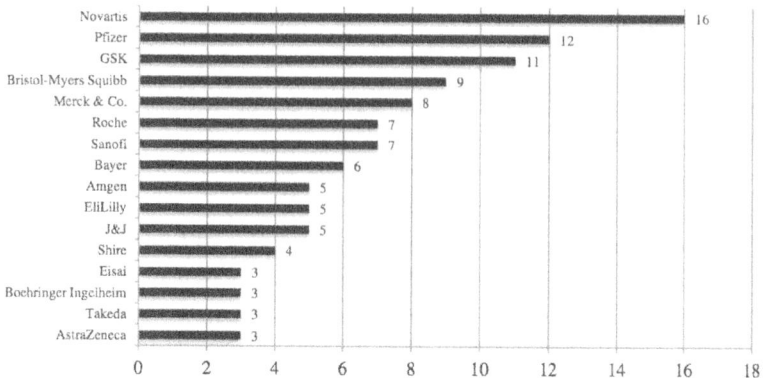

Figure 5: New molecular entities approved by FDA between 2001 and 2012 by major pharmaceutical companies
Source: Schuhmacher (2015), p.44

- *Increasing difficulty of offering benefits over existing treatments*
  The space for big medical breakthroughs is limited as many diseases can be already satisfactorily treated, even though the numbers of deaths from cancer, hard-to-treat diseases such as neurodegenerative or autoimmune diseases and deaths from cardiovascular diseases are still large[18] resulting in more technically complex investigations for new drug targets and respective clinical trials.

- *Stricter regulations by health authorities*
  Aside from the safety of a product, health authorities nowadays focus on whether a new drug is demonstrating benefits over existing treatment or not. This development is a result of the price development in the past, demographic changes and an ageing population, which is a major challenge for public health funds in the future. New drugs are usually very expensive when they come to market and are under patent protection, leading authorities to question whether the high price is justified, and a new treatment option must clearly demonstrate a benefit over the existing drugs. For example, countries like Germany and France have recently implemented changes in their health technology assessment (HTA) system that only allows price negotiations for drugs which demonstrate a benefit over existing treatment options. Drugs without a superior benefit will be paid at a lower level/put into the fixed price system or do not even

---

[18] Ding et al. (2014), p.8

get reimbursed.

- *Payers are gaining more power*
  Global ageing and the rise in chronic diseases are causing a steady increase in demand for health services. This development is accompanied by the actual trend of payers gaining more power in determining market access for drugs and imposing pressure on revenues and margins to be able to keep up with the rapidly rising demand of health services and fewer financial resources.

3.2 Measures Big Pharma is taking to address the challenges

In order to be able to compete in this ever-changing environment and to steer in the opposite direction of reduced R&D efficiency, pharmaceutical companies have responded by the following measures:

Increasing the number of projects in the R&D pipeline

In order to continuously fuel the R&D pipeline and to achieve the industry´s goal of launching 2-3 new molecular entities per year to meet their growth objectives[19], pharmaceutical companies have heavily invested from a resource and financial aspect into an increased number of R&D projects. Since 2001, the total number of projects listed in the pipelines of pharmaceutical companies worldwide has increased from 5,995 (2001) to 11,307 (2013).[20]

Reducing Costs of R&D

Between 2002 and 2011, the pharmaceutical and biotechnology sector has spent nearly US$1.1 trillion on R&D. However, as the R&D efficiency has decreased, pharmaceutical companies are now looking into ways to turn their R&D efforts into a more effective process by lowering costs at the same time. For example, in February 2011, Pfizer announced that it plans to cut its R&D costs by a third and a short time later Astra Zeneca made 2,200 scientists redundant. Simultaneously, Big Pharma has started to experiment with new R&D structures - GSK has set up several Centres of Excellence for Drug Discovery while Sanofi has re-organized its research department by underlying causes rather than disease areas.[21] In brief, a drop in R&D costs is generally related to a reduction in R&D personnel, a greater focus in project and portfolio management on project costs, and outsourcing of

---

[19] Schuhmacher (2015), p.45
[20] Schuhmacher (2015), p.57
[21] PwC (2012), p.24

research activities to low-cost countries to reduce operational and infrastructure costs. [22]

Actively Measuring Performance and Managing the Project Portfolio
The pharmaceutical industry has not only started to award greater attention to project costs and the project portfolio, but also towards the active management of the product portfolio. Managers are more acutely aware that the focus of R&D needs to change from late-stage development projects that may provide success in the near future to all phases of the drug development. Furthermore, portfolio decisions need to be based on medical need, technical feasibility, and commercial value.[23]

Opening R&D Towards External Innovation
On average, multinational pharmaceutical companies acquire 50% of their pipeline projects from external sources – either by in-licensing from biotech or pharmaceutical companies, collaborations (also with academia) or acquisitions.

---

[22] Schuhmacher (2015), p. 58
[23] Schuhmacher (2015), p. 60-61

4. Can Big Data overcome the innovation gap?

4.1 Big Data: Definition

The definition of Big Data varies in the scientific literature. According to the European Commission as described in ISO/IEC 2382-124, data is a

> "reinterpretable representation of information in a formalized manner, suitable for communication, interpretation or processing".

Data can either be created/authored by people or generated by machines/sensors, often as a "by-product".

The term "Big Data" refers to large amounts of different types of data produced with high velocity from high numbers of various types of sources.[25]

The available literature also often refers to the definition of Big Data by Gartner which is associated with the 3Vs[26]:

- **Volume:** Big Data consists of high amounts of data sets. According to the European Union, the world is generating 1.7 million billion bytes of data per minute. In other words, in average every man, woman and child on the planet is generating more than 6 megabytes per day.[27] As a consequence, massive amounts of data strain the capacity and capability of traditional data storage, management, and retrieval systems such as data warehouses. In fact, Big Data requires flexible and easily expandable data management solutions in order to source the total coverage of data available.

---

[24] International Organization for Standardization (2010)
[25] European Commission (2014), p.14
[26] Gartner (2013)
[27] European Commission (2) (2013)

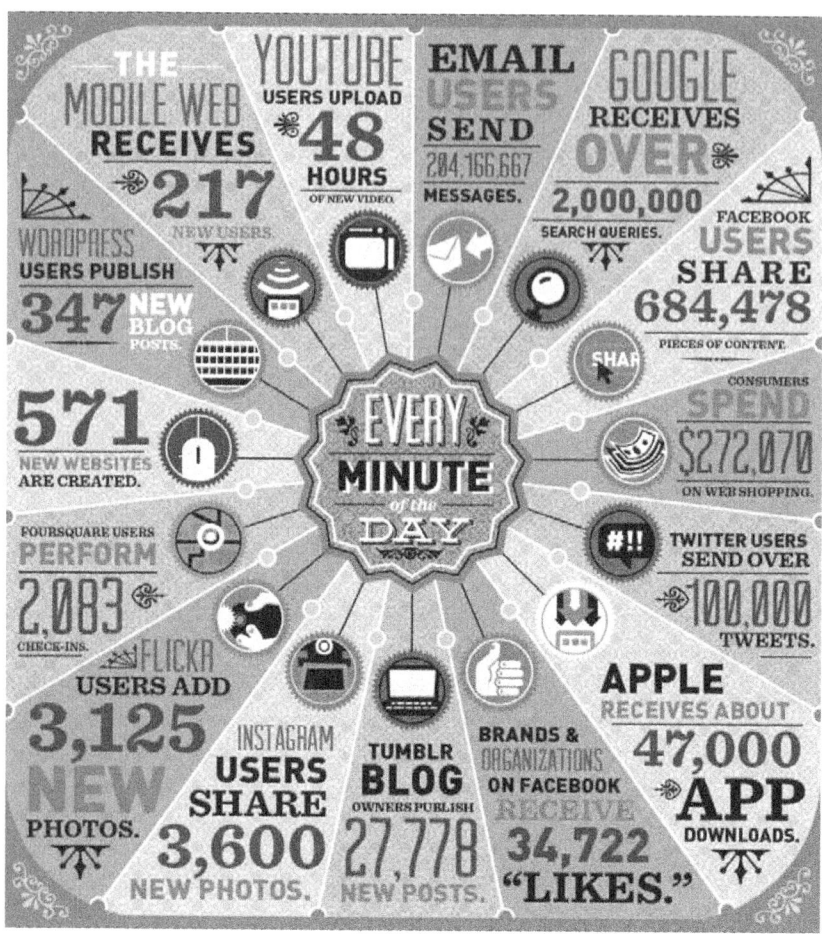

Figure 6: Volume and format of data created every minute online
Source: James (2012)

- **Velocity:** The second dimension concerns the dynamics of the volume of data and the speed of their creation.[28] Given recent advances in data management such as cloud computing, it is not only possible to store large amounts of data, but also to accumulate data in real-time and at rapid pace, or *velocity*.
- **Variety:** The potential of Big Data also lies in the different forms of data sets that are nowadays available – online and offline, structured and unstructured.

---

[28] Morabito (2015), p. VIII

Health devices and applications, genetics and genomics, social media, research and paper prescription are just a few of many examples of available data sources that produce a variety of different data sets.[29]

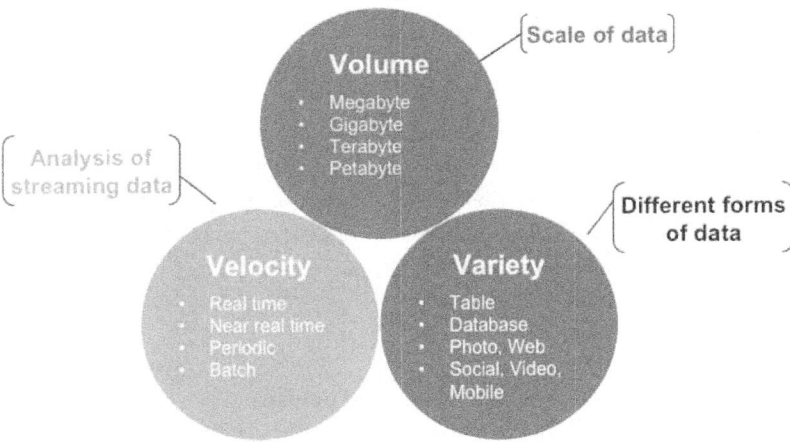

Figure 7: The Characteristics of Big Data – The 3 Vs
Source: Adapted from demos Europe (2014) and Morabito (2015)

Consequently, according to Gartner, Big Data is a high-volume, -velocity and -variety information asset that demands cost-effective, innovative forms of information processing for enhanced insight and decision-making.[30]

Some researchers have introduced a fourth characteristic, veracity, or 'data assurance' with regard to accuracy and truthfulness meaning that it is necessary to derive real insights from data sets. However, a lot of data experts contradict and say that veracity might be currently one of the major challenges of Big Data research, but not yet a characteristic of Big Data since quality issues of data sets are still of special concern. Finding ways to ensure error-free analytics and outcomes

[29] demos Europe (2014), p. 37-40
[30] Gartner (2013)

would be a huge step forward in making big data a more accurate source of information that enables informed decisions across sectors.[31]

Another term that has recently evolved in the data world is Smart Data, which is defined according to Iafrate as

> "the way in which different data sources (including Big Data) are brought together, correlated and analyzed to be able to feed decision-making and action processes."

Hence, in contrast to Big Data (in its technical approach itself) being concerned with data processing, Smart Data is concerned with analysis, value and integrating Big Data into business decision-making processes.[32]

In conclusion, Big Data are unstructured, highly complex, diverse and large data sets that have to be managed at high speed. Big Data itself is just an overwhelming data chaos that is difficult to handle. Analytics and analysis that extract the relevant and qualified data, also called Smart Data, are essential to derive any insights and value out of the steadily increasing data chaos.

4.2 Areas of use within the pharmaceutical industry

There is only very little literature available on Big Data and its use within the pharmaceutical industry. The literature that is available are articles or papers from leading consulting firms mainly focusing on the opportunities and challenges as well as strategies how to build a Big Data-oriented infrastructure to unlock its potential. However, as all publications were written by consulting firms or IT startups that mainly publish these sort of papers to symbolize thought leadership in this area with the aim to acquire new clients (e.g. pharma companies), the described opportunities are not proven and might make Big Data in some cases more promising than it is. A variety of challenges such as the patient's data privacy have yet to be overcome. Furthermore, there is not yet a clear and academic classification as to the extent and areas of use of Big Data for pharmaceutical companies. Nevertheless, given the scope of this study, the main areas below give an overview on the different application fields of Big Data based on the available publications to date, which will be used to classify and evaluate, in which areas the global top 5 pharma companies are active as per chapter 2.

---

[31] Raghupathi and Raghupathi (2014), p.4
[32] Iafrate (2015), p. 1 and 13

Main areas of Big Data potential according to published literature:

#1 -- **Drug discovery:**
- Enabling advanced search capabilities for analyzing millions of scientific publications, patents, diseases and clinical trial documents, helping researchers to discover potential areas for target drugs
- Identifying trial candidates in less time and a more cost-effective manner to accelerate their recruitment
- Uncovering unintended uses and thus new indications for well known products

#2 -- **Clinical trial management:**
- Enabling patient profiling by identifying the right candidates through analytics of demographic information and historical data, remote patient monitoring, reviewing previous clinical trial events as well as helping to identify potential side effects before they become known to the authorities
- Designing better inclusion and exclusion criteria to optimize the efficacy of clinical trials and their outcomes
- Targeting specific patient populations more effectively through combining data from genome sequencing, medical sensor[33] data and electronical medical records to understand how patients respond differently to treatments for a specific disease in order to develop more targeted medications for patients that share common characteristics

#3 -- **Safety and risk management (Pharmacovigilance):**
- Real world data gained by non-interventional studies to be used to disseminate relevant product information such as drug efficacy, adverse events to healthcare providers and payers to build brand awareness or to enhance product reimbursement in suitable cases
- Generating alerts about product safety issues by early warning signals coming from a range of unstructured data sources such as social media and Google search

---

[33] medical sensor – device worn by the patient which tracks physical changes during treatment

#4 -- Sales & marketing
- Spotting new, niche or underserved markets by analyzing information from social media, demographics, electronical medical records and other sources of data
- Analyzing the effectiveness of sales efforts and capturing the feedback received by the sales force during client visits to understand how to best create a competitive edge
- Understanding patient behavior through online analytics and data from remote sensor devices to gain greater insight into current patient behavior in order to design services targeted to different population or at risk patient groups with the overall aim to improve the efficacy of treatment (e.g. mobile app to remind the patient when to take his medication)[34,35,36]

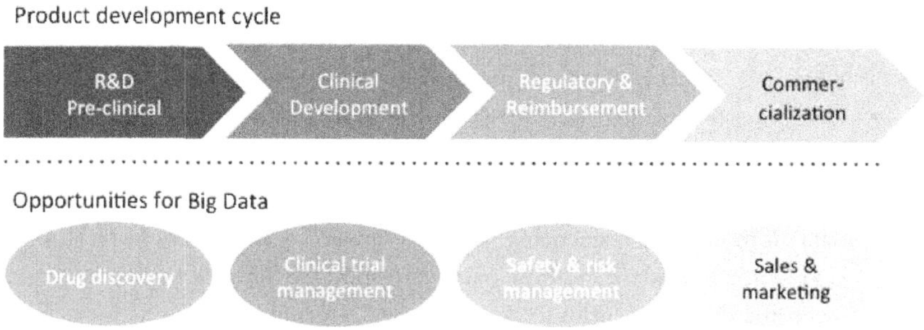

Product development cycle

| R&D Pre-clinical | Clinical Development | Regulatory & Reimbursement | Commercialization |

Opportunities for Big Data

Drug discovery | Clinical trial management | Safety & risk management | Sales & marketing

Figure 8: The opportunities for Big Data within the product value chain
Source: Own illustration (based on Morgon (2015) and Cattell et al. (2013))

The focus of this study will lie on how and to which extent pharmaceutical companies are using Big Data for the R&D process, namely drug discovery and clinical trial management.

4.3 Key hurdles for the acquisition and analysis of Big Data
Big Data is a promising research area with a lot of opportunities in the healthcare sector and for the pharmaceutical industry, in particular in the area of R&D. However, both the healthcare sector and the pharmaceutical industry are facing a num-

---
[34] Process Excellence Network (2014), p.3-9
[35] Cattell et al. (2013), p. 43-49
[36] Thomson Reuters (2013), p. 1-8

ber of challenges that first have to be overcome to unlock the potential of Big Data. Thereby, it is important to first of all understand that there are four distinct Big Data pools that have multiple owners, and that the different types of data are not shared among the various involved stakeholders (provider, payors, pharmaceutical companies, and academia).[37]

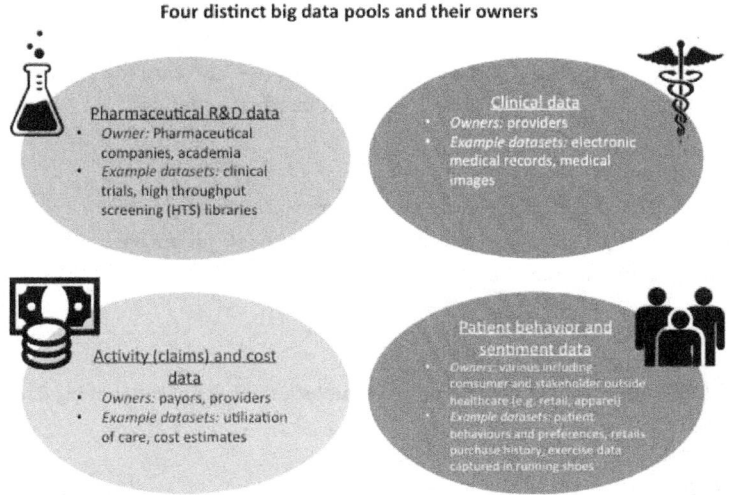

Figure 9: Four distinct data pools and their owners
Source: Own illustration; based on Cattell et al. (2013), p.4

Looking closer at the key hurdles of Big Data, we can distinguish between the challenges of data acquisition and data analysis:

---

[37] Cattell et al. (2013), p.4

Data acquisition:

Storage:
- Storage solutions are essential for managing large data volumes and delivering rapid results in a cost-effective manner. Organizations need fast, high-throughput connectivity solutions to reduce data bottlenecks, plus storage solutions that can balance performance, capacity, and cost.

Data management & transfer:
- Without the right IT infrastructure, analytic tools, visualization approaches, workflows, and interfaces, big data-driven insights are limited.

Connectivity:
- Integration of data pools and stakeholders are necessary to unlock the full potential of Big Data (clinicians, clinical researchers, pharmaceutical companies, healthcare policy-makers, etc.).

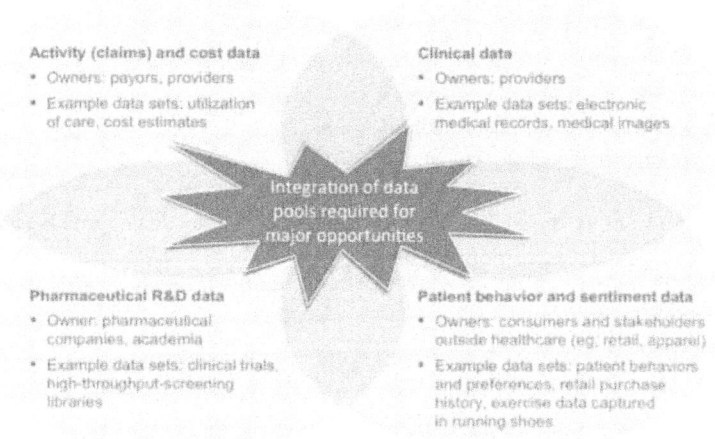

Figure 10: Required integration of data pools to unlock the full potential of Big Data
Source: Cattell et al. (2013), p.4

Interoperability:
- Data exchange schema and standards should permit data to be shared across clinicians, labs, hospitals, pharmacies and patients, regardless of the application or application vendor.

Data privacy:
- Personal data protection makes it difficult to access patient data and limits the availability of open data.

Data analysis:

Heterogeneity:
- Data is in most cases not only unstructured, but also generated or coded inconsistently which impedes the analysis of data that was generated by external sources.

Timeliness:
- The larger, more complex and unstructured the data set, the longer it will take to extract the insights. However, depending on the research question, the analysis of the data is required immediately to provide value; e.g. detecting a life-threatening complication in time.

Human resources:
- There is a rising need for staff with the required knowledge and expertise in the field of Big Data; e.g. statisticians to analyze the data, individuals with the technology skills to develop and manage big data systems and data managers who understand the nuances of data in great demand.

Harmonization:
- Different regulations from various countries make the global coordination and collaboration among researchers more difficult.[38,39]

4.4 Legal implications

The healthcare industry operates in a highly regulated space and technological faces a number of complex legal challenges, as it must comply with data protection

---

[38] Purdue University (2012), p. 9-14
[39] IMS Health (2012), p.8-11

and privacy rules. This chapter will focus on the 'spheres' of protection of healthcare data and legal requirements in the European Union.

'Spheres' of protection of healthcare information

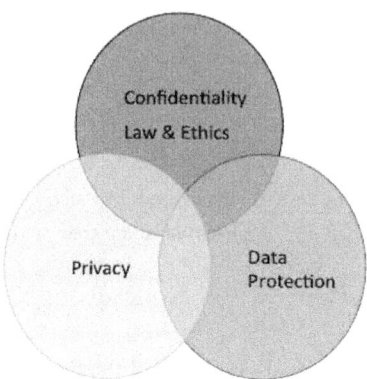

Figure 11: 'Spheres' of protection of healthcare information
Source: Eurosocap (x), p. 2

Privacy and the protection of personal data is a fundamental value. Article 8 of the Charter of Fundamental Rights of the European Union states:

Article 8 - Protection of personal data:

1. Everyone has the right to the protection of personal data concerning him or her.
2. Such data must be processed fairly for specified purposes and on the basis of the consent of the person concerned or some other legitimate basis laid down by law. Everyone has the right of access to data which has been collected concerning him or her, and the right to have it rectified.
3. Compliance with these rules shall be subject to control by an independent authority.[40]

---

[40] European Convention (2000), p. 10

Summarized, the principles include: fair information collection for a specific purpose, limitation to the specified purpose, accuracy, storage for no longer than necessary for the purpose, accessibility by the subject, and reasonable security.

The collection and use of health information engages the EU data protection law currently expressed in Directive 95/46/EC.

According to Directive 95/46/EC, data concerning health is sensitive personal data and therefore Member States shall prohibit the processing of health data – except where the data subject has given his explicit consent to the processing of those data (article 8) and has been made aware of the purposes and recipients of his personal data (article 10). Moreover, the prohibition is lifted where data processing is required for preventive medicine, medical diagnosis, provision of care or treatment or the management of health care services where processing is carried out by a healthcare professional or person subject to equivalent obligations of secrecy (article 8). Individual Member States may also specify exemptions from the prohibitions for reasons of substantial public interest so long as they provide suitable safeguards (article 8).

The principles of informed consent, privacy and data protection do also comply for clinical trials as per the EU Code of Clinical Trials (article 28) and are safeguarded in accordance to Directive 95/46/EC.[41]

The current Directive is due to be replaced by a Regulation as per the European Commission's decision in January 2012 to reform the data protection rules in the EU triggered amongst other reasons by the advances in technologies and the fact that the 27 EU Member Sates have implemented the 1995 rules differently, leading to divergences in enforcement, legal uncertainties and avoidable administrative costs. While the final Directive is still under discussion and a final agreement is earliest to be expected by the end of 2015, the first assumptions on the key changes can be made based on the published Regulation draft dated 19 December 2014[42]:

- The Regulation provides a more detailed definition of personal data concerning health, although in practice, it does not differ greatly on how health data is currently interpreted under the current Directive. But it also includes

---

[41] European Parliament (1995), p. 9 -17
[42] Council of the European Union (2014), p. 13ff

a definition of pseudonymous data which may, depending on the final version of the Regulation, give greater flexibility to the use of pseudonymous data.

- The position of the general prohibition on processing health data remains unchanged. Like the Directive, the prohibition does not prevent processing by a professional who is subject to secrecy for the purpose of preventive or occupational medicine, to assess employees, for medical diagnosis or provision of care, treatment or management of the healthcare system.

- Personal data can be processed for scientific purposes subject to appropriate conditions and safeguards set out in Member State or EU Law, and does not require consent from the data subject for each further processing.

- Processing data for health purposes is permitted for an important public interest ground especially where the processing is linked to a quality or cost-effectiveness benefit. Public health grounds permit the use of health data without the consent of individuals but such health data should not end up in the hands of third parties such as employers, insurance or banking companies. Moreover, the right to be forgotten provision will not require the erasure of health data processed for either public health reasons in the public interest or for scientific purposes.

- There are specific restrictions on profiling individuals in order to evaluate or analyze their health. Accordingly, a data protection impact assessment must be carried out in most instances of profiling to determine the risk to the rights and freedoms of the patient. However, an impact assessment is not mandatory where such processing is protected by professional secrecy and is administered, for example, by a healthcare professional.[43]

Putting the fundamental right of privacy and data protection into perspective by comparing it with the principles and characteristic of Big Data, it becomes obvious that current law interferes with the methodological approach of Big Data:

---

[43] Hordern (2015), p. 2-3

Big Data and issues for privacy

Principles of data protection law	Big Data
Personal data can be only gathered for a legitimate purpose	Collection of all available data for as many purposes as possible
Aim of processing and using as little personal data as possible	Unlimited use and processing of data
Health data is sensitive personal data and processing is prohibited without explicit consent	Sensitive data protection laws hinder scientific insights and advances in research
Transparency of data processing for data subjects	No transparency given the unstructured and multi-purpose nature of Big Data
Data management and techniques have to be in line with data protection laws	Data management and techniques aim to overcome technical barriers in order to gain maximal insights

Figure 12: Big Data and privacy issues
Source: Own illustration, based on Petri (2015), p. 12-13

As a conclusion, while the European Commission has understood the legal implications for Big Data and is currently in the process of discussing the current Regulation draft with the Member States, there is still a long way to go until data privacy laws will be lifted in a manner that allows unlimited use and collection of health data for multiple purposes, if at all, to unlock the full value of Big Data. The currently on-going discussions with the Member States that have already delayed the finalization and publication of the announced Regulation are a sign of how sensitive the topic of data privacy is. It becomes obvious that it will be also necessary to change mind sets and build trust in today´s available IT advances that allow much more secure data processing than, for example, a decade ago, in order to ensure a successful implementation of the Regulation within the European Union.

5. Online research: Use and impact of Big Data for R&D among top 5 pharmaceutical companies

5.1 Methodology

To examine how active and advanced the global top pharmaceutical companies are (based on the key questions in chapter 2), an online research has been conducted. Thereby the following publically available sources and research methodologies have been applied:

1. Company Website:
The company websites of all five identified pharma companies (Novartis, Pfizer, Sanofi, Roche, Merck & Co) were screened by using the search strings "big data", "big data AND R&D" and "big data AND research and development" within the search function of the homepage. The search results that included further insights on Big Data for R&D were selected.

2. Google research:
Using the search strings ""name of pharmaceutical company" AND "big data"", the web was screened for publications, announcements or other publicly available information of any of the top 5 pharmaceutical companies with regard to Big Data and R&D in English and German language. Any hits on Big Data congresses were ignored as they are listed in category 3 (see below). Given the fact that Big Data technologies are a fast moving topic, only search results that were posted within the last three years (July 2012 – July 2015) were taken into account.

3. International and regional congresses on Big Data and the pharmaceutical industry:
A Google search was conducted to compile a list of all established international and regional congresses on Big Data in general, specific conferences on Big Data for the pharmaceutical industry and health innovation congresses (please see appendix 2 and 3 for used search words and results). The congress websites, agendas/programs, abstracts and publications were screened by using the following methodology:
1. Have representatives of the top 5 pharmaceutical companies participated in any of the identified congresses?

2. If so, what are the titles of the presentations/speeches? Are there abstracts or a more detailed program description available?
3. Do the titles of the presentations and abstracts give any insights on Big Data projects and strategies for R&D?

5.2 Results

5.2.1 Novartis

1. Company Website

The research on the company website (www.novartis.com) itself showed two results (as of July 2015):

Source	Insights
Surfing the Wave of Big Data Analytics[44] (Article posted on 27 October 2013 by Tia O´Brien)	• Success story of a collaborative effort by Novartis and the Necker Children´s Hospital-Imagine Foundation in Paris applying DNA sequencing technology and analytics to detect the cause of a kidney cancer called focal segmental glomerulosclerosis (FSGS).
A normal life is extraordinary[45] (Post including Youtube video on company website published on 19 May 2015)	• As part of the mission of Novartis to dedicate efforts and knowledge to search for treatments and cures for long, healthy lives, the company also mentions Big Data analysis as part of their research pathways to work towards this goal.

2. Google research

Using the search string ""Novartis" AND "big data"" has shown eleven results of interest. News about Novartis that have been published by different online media outlets are only mentioned once if the content did not differ from other publications.

Source	Insights
The patient Big data challenge: Big Data & Analytics for Pharma conference (Blog on Treato Blog published on 18 June 2013 by Yaron Landow)[46]	• The Blog mentions the presentation of Susan Massaro, Head of Economics at Novartis, on the difficulty in accessing large amounts of quality data at the Big Data & Analytics for Pharma Conference in Philadelphia. "Finding the right patient, the right treatment, at the right time"

---

[44] O´Brien (2013)
[45] Novartis (2015)

	has been one of the major topics. Massaro also spoke about how Novartis is accessing data from patient registries and self-created and closed patient forums to gain more insights into clinical trial monitoring criteria such as adverse events. However, Novartis is now posing the question how to find Big Patient Data – a more scalable solution to enable them to access large amounts of this quality data.
Lilly, Novartis and Pfizer sign up to improve ClinicalTrials.gov (Article on FierceBiotech-IT.com published on 24 November 2013 by Nick Paul Taylor)[47]	• Novartis, Pfizer and Elli Lilly have been tasked by the US government to help improve ClinicalTrials.gov in order to make it more effective at matching patients to studies. The three pharma companies are asked to add a machine-readable "target health profile" for 50 clinical trials.
Novartis extends leadership in clinical trial data transparency, reinforcing its support of clinical research and innovation (Company press release published on 26 February 2014)[48]	• Novartis announced additional steps to extend its clinical trial data transparency by launching the ideaPoint portal that allows researchers access to patient level data on newly approved innovative medicines in the United States and EU in 2014. • Furthermore the company announced that it is committed to enhancing Clinical Study Report summaries for all new pivotal studies to include easy-to-understand consumer language and additional interpretation of data as of the end of 2014.
Der Mann, der den Krebs mit viel Geld besiegen will (Interview in Die Welt with Joseph Jimenez, CEO Novartis, by Nando Sommerfeldt and Holger Zschäpitz on 24 April 2014)[49]	• On the occasion of the acquisition of GSK´s oncology business by Novartis, Joseph Jimenez gives an outlook on the company´s future efforts in R&D for oncology and other therapeutic areas including the potential of Big Data for clinical trials. • According to Jimenez, Big Data has the potential to soon understand the full genetic composition of patients that will allow developing more targeted drugs and conducting more efficient and less time-consuming clinical trials. • However, Jimenez regards ethics and privacy laws as a major barrier for Big Data and emphasizes the benefits of having access to anonymous data in order to leverage scientific findings.

---

[46] Landow (2013)
[47] Taylor (2013)
[48] Novartis (2014)
[49] Sommerfeldt and Zschäpitz (2014)

Broad and Novartis Keep Up with Big Data (Article on Bio-ITWorld.com published on 15 May 2014 by Matt Luchette)[50]	• Summary of a joint presentation of Andrea DeSouza, from the Broad Institute, and Anne Mai Wassermann, from Novartis, on new technologies to squeeze meaning from researchers´ vast amount of data at the Bio-IT World Conference & Expo. • Wassermann presents the company´s suite of three visualization tools: HTS-Explorer, Chemotography, and Con-Tour. The tools work synergistically to help researchers visualize data and identify promising drug candidates.

Big Pharma heiratet Big Data - Was haben Novartis und Google vor? (Article published in Blick.ch on 16 July 2014 by Guido Schätti and Jenni Thier)[51]	• Novartis´eye care division Alcon has entered into an agreement with a division of Google Inc. to in-license its "smart lens" technology for all ocular medical uses. Google provides Alcon with the opportunity to develop and commercialize Google's "smart lens" technology with the potential to:
	   ○ Help diabetic patients manage their disease by providing a continuous, minimally invasive measurement of the body's glucose levels via a "smart contact lens" which is designed to measure tear fluid in the eye and connects wirelessly with a mobile device;
	   ○ For people living with presbyopia who can no longer read without glasses, the "smart lens" has the potential to provide accommodative vision correction to help restore the eye's natural autofocus on near objects in the form of an accommodative contact lens or intra-ocular lens as part of the refractive cataract treatment.

Covance and Novartis team up with eyes on Big Data (Article on Fiercecro.com published on 13 October 2014 by Damian Garde)[52]	• Novartis has initiated a collaboration with Covance, a drug development service company, to expand the Novartis Institutes for Biomedical Research´s (NIBR) existing clinical data warehouse and to develop ways to quickly integrate and analyse large volumes of results from pre-clinical and clinical studies.
Creating Flexible Big Data Solutions for Drug Discovery (Article on datanami.com published on 19 January 2015)[53]	• Article on David Tester, an application architect at Novartis Institutes for Biomedical Research, who has developed both a workflow and integration solution in order to address the two major challenges of Next Generation Sequencing (NGS): ○ NGS requires workflow tools that are robust enough

---

[50] Luchette (2014)
[51] Schätti and Thier (2014)
[52] Garde (2014)
[53] datanami (2015)

	to process vast amounts of raw NGS data yet flexible enough to keep up with quickly changing research techniques. o NGS requires a way to meaningfully integrate data from Novartis with data from large external organizations (e.g. 1000 Genomes, Cancer Genome Atlas, etc.).
Drug Discovery in the Era of Big Data (Slides by Gregory McAllister published on 19 January 2015)[54]	• Presentation explaining Novartis' drug discovery strategy driven by the Novartis Institutes for BioMedical Research (NIBR). • Named current and future hurdles as increasing data size, dimensionality of data and complexity. • An open source and multi-dimensional data management system is required for large scale analytics.
Novartis Relies on MapR for Flexible Big Data Solutions for Drug Discovery (Novartis Customer Brief published by MapR Technologies in 2015)[55]	• The Novartis Institutes for BioMedical Research uses the data system called MapR to integrate diverse datasets from external institutions to accelerate drug research in the field of Next Generation Sequencing (NGS). The system also facilitates the interactions between computer scientists and life scientists.
AWS Case Study: Novartis (Case study on AmazonWebServices.com, last updated in 2015)[56]	• Novartis case study on a project run in 2013 that involved virtually screening 10 million compounds against a common cancer target in less than a week. Novartis calculated that it would take 50,000 cores (multicore processor) and close to a $40 million investment if they wanted to run the experiment internally. Partnering with Cycle Computing and Amazon Web Services (AWS), Novartis built a platform leveraging Amazon Simple Storage Service (Amazon S3), Amazon Elastic Block Store (Amazon EBS), and four Availability Zones. The project ran across 10,600 Spot Instances (approximately 87,000 compute cores) and allowed Novartis to conduct 39 years of computational chemistry in 9 hours for a cost of $4,232. Out of the 10 million compounds screened, three were successfully identified.

---

[54] McAllister (2011)
[55] MapR (2015)
[56] Amazon Web Services (2015)

3. Congresses

The screening of websites/abstracts/programs of Big Data congresses in general or specifically for the pharmaceutical industry has shown seven results on Novartis and R&D:

Name of congress	Insights
Big Data Events for Pharma (Google search strings: "big data congress pharma"; "big data conference pharma"; "big data summit pharma")	
Big Data in Pharma 12-13 May 2014 (London, UK)	• **Presentation: Leveraging Big Data To Study Comparative Effectiveness Research (CER): A Case Example in Multiple Sclerosis** *(Niklas Bergvall, Senior Director, Global HEOR Neuroscience)* • **Presentation: Leveraging Existing Data From Legacy Clinical Trials** *(Pantaleo Nacci, Head Statistical Reporting)* • **Shared Presentation: Lessons Learned So Far! Understanding Big Data And Its Uses For The Pharmaceutical World** *(Pantaleo Nacci, Head Statistical Reporting)*

Oxford Global Annual Pharmaceutical IT Congress 23-24 September 2015 (London, UK)	• Speakers (presentations to be confirmed):
	   o Dimitrios Georgiopoulos, Chief Scientific Officer UK
	   o Philippe Marc, Global Head of Preclinical Informatics, Novartis Institutes for Biomedical Research
	   o Eric Martin, Computational Chemistry
	   o Abhimanyu Verma, Head Real World Evidence & Big Data – R&D Informatics

Oxford Global Pharmaceutical IT World Asia Congress 25-26 March 2014 (Singapore)	• Speakers:
	   o Stephen Elms, Head of Automation & IT, Biopharmaceutical Operations Singapore
	   o Dinesh Pillaipakkamnatt, Global Head, Central Analytics Function

Fleming Europe Pharma Exabyte 27-28 May 2015 (Berlin, Germany)	• Speakers: Edward Oakeley, Basel Head, Next Generation Sequencing Technologies
Bio Data World Congress 21-22 October 2015 (Cambridge, USA)	• **Presentation: The current and future status of ultra-long read sequencing studies** *(Edward Oakeley, Basel Head, Next Generation Sequencing Technologies)*

Big Data in Pharma 2015 17 June 2015 (London, UK)	• **Presentation: Big Data in Clinical Trials: An Experience in Vaccines** *(Pantaleo Nacci, Head of Statistical Reporting)*
Bio IT World Conference EXPO 21-23 April 2015 (Boston, USA)	• **Workshop: Predicitive Anayltics** -- Instructors among other representatives (Exaptve, GNS Healthcare, Tamr): *Mark Burfoot – Global Head, Knowledge Office, Novartis Institutes for BioMedical Research*

5.2.2 Pfizer:
1. Company Website:
The research on the company website (www.pfizer.com) itself showed three results:

Source	Insights
Humedica and Pfizer Form Strategic Alliance (Company press release published on 20 December 2012)[57]	• Pfizer and Humedica agreed on a multi-year strategic alliance to jointly advance capabilities to derive insights from real world data by leveraging Humedica's expertise in gathering and normalizing de-identified healthcare data from disparate systems and Pfizer's experience in researching, developing and commercializing medicines to prevent and treat health conditions.
Pfizer US Medical, Scientific, Patient and Civic Organization Funding Report Q3 2013 (Company report published on 26 November 2013)[58]	• Pfizer US has provided Health Affairs with a fund of $5,000 for a 'Proposal for Thematic Issue on the Impact of Big Data on Health Care and Health Research'.
CliniWorks Forms a Strategic Alliance with Pfizer to Develop a Population Health Management Platform with Advanced Analytics and Patient Care Capabilities (Company press release published on 7 July 2014)[59]	• Strategic alliance between CliniWorks subsidiary in Israel (CliniWorks Israel) and Pfizer to develop a population health management platform solution that leverages CliniWorks' technologies in disparate data aggregation and Natural Language Processing (which interprets free text information) of de-identified healthcare data and aims to enable large medical groups and integrated delivery systems institutions to deliver near real-time and more efficient and effective quality healthcare. Furthermore, it is supposed to improve patient engagement or

---

[57] Pfizer (2012)
[58] Pfizer (2013)
[59] Pfizer (2014)

	activation reaching the Centers for Medicare and Medicaid Triple Aim. • The development work will be partially supported by a grant from the Bird Foundation. [60]

2. Google Research:

Using the search string ""Pfizer" AND "big data"" and screening the hits for insights regarding R&D has shown five results of interest:

Source	Insights
Pfizer Swaps Out ETL for Data Virtualization Tools (Article on TechTarget.com by Nicole Laskowski published in February 2013)[61]	• The Business Information Systems unit of Pfizer has moved from ETL (extract, transform, load) process to data virtualization tools to minimize cost and time issues, and maximize quality.
Pfizer Seeks Insights Into Big Data Analysis, Personalized Medicine Through Optum Labs (Article in The Pink Sheet by Gregory Twachtman, published on 24 February 2014)[62]	• Pfizer has started a collaboration with Optum Labs focusing on gaining insights into personalized medicine and testing new methodologies for analyzing real-world data. • Optum Labs was launched in January 2013 as collaboration between Optum, the research business of UnitedHealth Group.Co, and the Mayo Clinic with the goal to link claims data with clinical health records in a way that allows researchers to analyze the data in order to find ways to improve outcomes and reduce the cost of health care delivery. Pfizer was among seven organizations that were announced as new members in the research collaboration.
Pfizer Connects Dots To Deliver Better Treatments (Article on InformationWeek.Com by Doug Henschen published on 2 April 2014)[63]	• Pfizer is using the Precision Medicine Analytics Ecosystem that connects the dots among genomic, clinical trial, and electronic medical record data to identify opportunities to quickly deliver new drugs for specific patient populations (mentioned example Xalkori for lung cancer patients that have a mutation in their ALK

---

[60] BIRD is an acronym for Israel-U.S. Binational Industrial Research and Development. The BIRD Foundations´s mission is to stimulate, promote and support industrial R&D of mutual benefit to the U.S. and Israel.
[61] Laskowski (2013)
[62] Twachtman (2015)
[63] Henschen (2014)

	gene). The ecosystem program consists of three different components:
	    o tranSMART, an open source data management system to combine genomic data sets from internal and external sources.
	    o Clinical Cloud, a cloud-based clinical data repository, enables Pfizer to aggregate data from different companies to acquire additional clinical data.
	• An EMR (electronic medial record) component that contains hundreds of millions of anonymized data sets.

How Pfizer Is Using Big Data To Power Patient Care (Guest post on Forbes.Com by Geno Germano, Group President, Global Innovative Pharma Business, Pfizer posted on 17 February, 2015)[64]	• Blog post on how big data research will advance clinical trial research and ultimately enable faster completion of clinical trials and thus more effective and preventive care for patients. • Advances in detecting fibromyalgia through Pfizer's large Electronic Medical Record database of de-identified patient data and the creation of a model to help clinicians identify patients that might be suffering from fibromyalgia earlier so patients can receive more effective care. • Pfizer is working with a big data company to assess the value of data in understanding the obesity epidemic and how it may inform the development of medicine.

Pfizer: From Data-Supported to Data-Enabled
(Forum Post in Open Forum by Anisha Baghudana on 14 April, 2015)[65]
	• At Pfizer, the company's Big Data strategy sits with the Global Data Management (GDM) team. GDM acts as a shared centralized resource for all functions - mainly, research and development (R&D), finance and procurement, commercial, manufacturing and corporate.
	• In the last three years, Pfizer has started making a more conscious choice to use data analytics in more upstream business functions like the R&D and innovation process. Particularly, Pfizer is directing big data towards the following:
	    o How to tailor treatments for small patient populations while staying highly profitable
	    o How to bring drugs to market faster, thus cutting development costs
	    o How to develop more efficacious drugs

---

[64] Germano (2015)
[65] Baghudana (2014)

	- Pfizer's strategy – 3 Cs: Connect, Collect, Comprehend:
	  ○ *Connect:* Pfizer is sharing clinical trial results on data-sharing platforms following the trend by GSK and Sanofi to post trial results on ClinicalDataStudyRequest.com so that disparate sources of data across companies could become connected.
	  ○ *Collect:* Pfizer's Precision Medicine Analytics Ecosystem looks for non-obvious patterns between genomic data, clinical trials data and de-identified medical records to draw insights.
	  ○ *Comprehend:* Pfizer is already capturing value from the data transparency movement and efficient, targeted processes for collecting data. It has developed drugs (e.g. Xalkori) for chronic conditions that in the past took much longer to diagnose.

3. Congresses

The screening of websites/abstracts/programs of big data congresses in general or specifically for the pharmaceutical industry has shown 15 results on Pfizer and R&D:

Name of congress	Insights
Big Data Events for Pharma (Google search strings: "big data congress pharma"; "big data conference pharma"; "big data summit pharma")	
Pharma Data Analytics 29 September–1 October 2014 (Brussels, Belgium)	- Gerhard Noelken, Business IT Lead, member of congress advisory board
Big Data & Analytics for Pharma Summit 4-5 November 2015 (Philadelphia, USA)	- Speaker (presentation to be confirmed): Catherine Marshall, Director, Information Strategy & Analytics
Big DIP Europe 27-29 January 2015 (London, UK)	- Chairman at the Congress: Josephine A. Sallono, Vice President, Outcomes & Evidence, Global Health and Value
Big DIP USA 22-24 September 2014 (Boston, USA)	- Sample speaker: Marc Berger, Vice President, Real World Data & Analytics

Oxford Global Annual Pharmaceutical IT Congress
 23-24 September 2015
 (London, UK)
	• Speakers (presentations to be confirmed):
	    o Marc Berger, Vice President, Real World Data & Analytics
	    o Gerhard Noelken, Global Business IT Lead for Pharmaceutical Science
	    o Sergio H. Rotstein, Director, Research Business Technology
	    o Q&A: Marc Berger, Vice President, Real World Data & Analytics

Oxford Global Pharmaceutical IT World Asia Congress
 25-26 March 2014
 (Singapore)
	• Speakers:
	    o Jay Bergeron, Director, Translational and Bioinformatics
	    o Gerhard Noelken, Global Business IT Lead for Pharmaceutical Science

Big Data in Clinical Development 2015 7-8 October 2015 (Washington DC, USA)	• **Chair's Introductory Remarks: Leveraging human genetics in drug discovery** *(Dr. Morten Sogaar, VP & Head Enterprise Scientific Technology Operations)* • **Presentation: Disruptive Innovations in Clinical Trials, EHR Reuse** *(David Isom, Global Head, R&D Information and Strategy Analytics)*
Cambridge Healthtech Institute's Seventh Annual Integrated Pharma Informatics & Data Science 16- 18 February 2015 (San Francisco, USA)	• **Presentation: Using Informatics to Enable Precision Medicine in Oncology** *(Susie Stephens, Senior Director, Oncology & West Coast IT, Pfizer)*
Fleming Europe Pharma Exabyte 27-28 May 2015 (Berlin, Germany)	• Speaker: Jerry Lanfear, Head of Research Business Technologies
Marcus Evans Annual Pharma Data Analytics 18-19 November 2014 (Philadelphia, USA)	• Speaker: Aaron Galaznik, MD, MBA, Senior Director, Real World Data and Analytics, Global Health and Value
Bio IT World Conference & EXPO 21-23 April 2015 (Boston, USA)	*Clinical & Translational Informatics* • **Presentation: Technology Framework to Operationalize Biomarker-Focused Clinical Research** *(Brenda Yanak, Ph.D., Director, Precision Medicine Leader, Clinical Innovation)* *Data Visualization and Exploration Tools* • **Presentation: Towards an Open Source Suite to**

	Bridge the Gap between Plate-Based Screening and Results *(Peter Henstock, Ph.D., Senior Principal Scientist, Research Business Technology Group)*
	Collaborations and Open Access Innovations • Presentation: Imitation and Disruption: Impact on Open Source Software Success in the Life Sciences *(Jay Bergeron, Director, Translational and Bioinformatics)* • Panel discussion: Finding Innovation in Collaboration Environments: Documentum SharePoint, Veeva, and Tigers, Oh My! *(Instructor among other representatives from Biogen, AstraZeneca, J&J: Jay Bergeron, Direcor, Translational & Bioinformatics)*
Bio Data World Congress 21-22 October 2015 (Cambridge, USA)	• Presentation: NGS and the discovery of causative genes for pain *(Dr. Ciara Vangjeli, Associate Director and Senior Applied Geneticist)*
Cambridge's Healthtech Institute's Biomarker & Diagnostics World Congress 5-7 May 2015 (Philadelphia, USA)	• Presentation: Using Clinical and Real World Data for Biomarker Discovery in Precision Medicine *(Joan Sopczynski, Ph.D., Senior Manager, Predictive Informatics, Business Insights, R&D Business Technology)*
Real World Evidence & Data Partnerships Summit 14-15 October 2014 (Bethesda, USA)	• Pharma Case Study: Leveraging Real World Data to Inform Decision-Making on a Timely Basis *(Marc Berger, Vice President, Real World Data & Analytics)*
Predictive Analytics World for Healthcare 27 September–1 October 2015 (Boston, USA)	• Case Study: Crowdsourcing Predictive Analytics to Enhance Clinical Trial Design *(Scott Jelinski, Principal Research Scientist)*

5.2.3 Sanofi

1. Company Website
The research on the company website of Sanofi (www.sanofi.com) showed one result.

Source	Insights

Clinical Trials: Our Data Sharing Commitments (Company statement, 2015)[66]	• Sanofi believes that making clinical trial data available to the research community promises to advance science and medicine, contribute to improvements in public health and improve knowledge about and trust in pharmaceutical drug development.
	• The pharmaceutical industry as a whole demonstrated its support for sharing of clinical data when in July 2013, the members of PhRMA and EFPIA developed and endorsed a set of Principles for Responsible Sharing of Clinical Trial Data. They include five commitments:
	  o Enhancing Data Sharing with Researchers
	  o Enhancing Public Access to Clinical Study Information
	  o Sharing Results with Patients who Participate in Clinical Trials
	  o Certifying Procedures for Sharing Clinical Trial Information
	  o Reaffirming Commitments to Publish Clinical Trial Results

2. Google research
Using the search string ""Sanofi" AND "big data"" and screening the hits for insights regarding R&D has shown five results of interest:

Source	Insights
Sanofi partners with 'Big Data' firm to enhance translational medicine (Post on ClinDev.EU published on 1 May 2013)[67]	• Sanofi and NextBio have announced a multi-year collaboration to incorporate patient omics[68] and clinical data into Sanofi's drug research and development, as part of Sanofi's Translational Medicine for Patients (TM4P) program.

---

[66] Sanofi (2015)
[67] ClinDev.EU (2013)
[68] The English-language neologism omics informally refers to a field of study in biology ending in -omics, such as genomics, proteomics or metabolomics.

	• NextBio will provide Sanofi with the NextBio Clinical platform for aggregation, standardization and analysis of patient clinical data, next generation sequencing (NGS) and other molecular data across public data sources, clinical trials and hospital partners.
Sanofi Will Share Clinical Trial Data, But There Is A Caveat (Article on Forbes.Com by Ed Silverman published on 2 January 2014)[69]	• Sanofi has committed to release its clinical trial data and will join an effort begun by GSK to establish a website (ClinicalstudyDataRequest.com) where researchers can request study information. • Sanofi will make available trial data and related documents, including clinical study reports, for studies in human that were submitted to US and European regulators and the product must have been approved by both agencies – on or after January 1, 2014. • Although the company says it will continue to submit for publication the results from all company-sponsored clinical studies, regardless of the study outcome, trial data for older prescription drugs and vaccines will not be made available to researchers.
Big Pharma Opens Up Its Big Data (Article in MIT Technology Review by Arlene Weintraub published on 21 July 2014)[70]	• After GlaxoSmithKline (GSK) has started the transparency trend of making available detailed data from its clinical trials, Sanofi has also put its trial results on ClinicalStudyDataRequest.com and has posted three prostate cancer trials on Project Data Sphere, a pharma-supported site aimed at using data sharing to speed up the development of new cancer cures. According to Philip Huang, vice president of strategic planning and operations for Sanofi: "The next step will be to unify the procedures followed in clinical trials." • In September 2012, Sanofi, GSK, and Roche helped found TransCelerate BioPharma, a non-profit organization that creates standards for collecting and reporting clinical-trial data.
Interview with Brian Ellerman (Interview posted on Phacilitate.co.uk ahead of the Phacilitate Big data Leader´s Forum 2014)[71]	• Brian Ellerman, Head of Technology Scouting and Information Science Innovation and being responsible for coordinating and leading development of R&D´s global digital strategy emphasizes that harnessing Big Data in R&D is a major priority for Sanofi and the in-

---

[69] Silverman (2014)
[70] Weintraub (2014)
[71] Phacilitate.co.uk (2014)

	dustry. • Big Data in the clinical trial area bringing together all types of unusual and disparate data and the area of 'digital medicine' or 'digital health' driven by the quantified 'self data' generated by wearable devices are of particular interest. • The biggest challenges are data maintenance and transformation while looking at clinical trials data from different companies.
IBM Watson Speeds Drug Research (Article on InformationWeek.com by Doug Henschen published on 28 August 2014)[72]	• IBM announced that drug giants Johnson & Johnson and Sanofi are working with Watson to speed research initiatives. Johnson & Johnson is collaborating with the Discovery Advisor team to teach Watson to read and understand scientific papers that detail clinical trial outcomes used in evaluating treatments. The collaborators are hoping to accelerate drug comparative-effectiveness studies. Sanofi hopes to speed drug re-purposing, which is the discovery of alternative indications for existing drugs.

3. Congresses

The screening of websites/abstracts/programs of big data congresses in general or specifically for the pharmaceutical industry has shown four results on Sanofi and R&D:

Name of congress	Insights
Big Data Events for Pharma (Google search strings: "big data congress pharma"; "big data conference pharma"; "big data summit pharma")	
Big DIP Europe 27-29 January 2015 (London, UK)	• **Presentation: Innovative Partnering for Holistic Results: Who, Why & How** *(Charles Gerrits, Vice President, Early Patient & Medical Perspectives)*

Oxford Global Annual Pharmaceutical IT Congress
23-24 September 2015
(London, UK)
	• Speakers (presentations to be confirmed):
	  o James Connelly, Global Head, Research Data Management
	  o Brian Ellerman, Head of Technology Scouting and Information Science Innovation
	  o Charles Gerrits, Innovative Patient-Centric Endpoints and Solutions

---

[72] Henschen (2) (2014)

Big Data in Clinical Development 2015 7-8 October 2015 (Washington DC, USA)	• Presentation: How the cloud is overcoming the problems of distance and data size in clinical trials *(Rhett Alden, Senior Director, Cloud)* • Presentation: The value of Big Data: how analytics differentiates winners *(Dr. William Daley, VP, Medical Affairs, Aging, Business Development & Licensing)* • Presentation: Finding the data: patients as partners in medicines development *(Francis Rienzo, Vice President of Partners in Patient Health)*
Real World Evidence & Data Partnerships Summit 14-15 October 2014 (Bethesda, USA)	• Presentation: Where Rubber Hits the Road: Customer-Driven Evidence – Real World Data for Business Decisions *(William L. Daley, Vice President, Business Development & Licensing, Sanofi)*

5.2.4 Roche

1. Company Website

The research on the company website (www.roche.com) itself showed six results:

Source	Insights

Extracting Value From the Data Deluge
(Story in Roche media store, posted on 28 February 2014)[73]
	• Bryan Roberts, Global Head of pRED Informatics highlights the challenges of Big Data in R&D and presents solutions to overcome these:
	  • "Yet to make effective decisions through the course of a drug discovery and development project, we must combine the claims from the scientific literature with external data and Roche internal data of many kinds such as high throughput screening, toxicology, target selectivity, metabolism and pharmacokinetics, in vitro and in vivo efficacy, imaging, etc. Add to these the complexity at the individual genetic level—for example, polymorphisms that affect the way in which drugs interact with their target biological molecules or are metabolized and eliminated from the body—, then one really starts to appreciate the Big Data challenge in R&D, namely how to make data actionable to support key decisions, thus maximizing the chances of success."
	  • "Importantly, addressing the Big Data challenge in

---

[73] Roche (1) (2014)

	R&D requires a multidisciplinary approach where biologists, computer scientists, toxicologists, statisticians, chemists, and many others need to work in a highly collaborative way."
	• Information Technology will help with the integration of data from many sources and formats, as well as new approaches to visualize and explore very large information landscapes. "Analysis algorithms will also allow scientists to extract meaning from massively complex data. Finally, novel human-computer interfaces will enable multidisciplinary teams to interact with their data more meaningfully, enabling effective decisions when moving projects forward."
Big Data (Webpage with embedded YouTube video, published on 10 June 2014)[74]	• Roche has always been in the business of generating data and based on that delivering innovative medicines and diagnostic tests to patients. • The amount of data is exploding and Roche invests particular attention in devising systems that allow extraction of information from the data, sharing within project teams and deriving meaningful knowledge that drives the drug discovery process

Big Data – Revealing the Unseen (Feature in Roche media online store, posted on 21 July 2014)[75]	• Roche uses 'Big Data' as an umbrella term for methods and technologies that enable to process vast amounts of data.
	• At present, nine big data projects are under way at Roche and more pilot requests are under review. "We need to be aware that big data technology only starts to emerge. Looking at all sectors as a whole, 85 percent of all projects and pilots do not deliver any insight that can be converted into a direct business benefit," says Simon Ulrich, Head of Business Intelligence & Master Data Management in Pharma Informatics. Project examples are:
	    o A joint Global Product Strategy, Medical Affairs and Product Development project is aiming to use data which has been generated outside of controlled clinical studies. These records could still be relevant to demonstrating the effectiveness of medicines.
	    o Pilot projects in pRED are trying to find out,

---

[74] Roche (2) (2014)
[75] Roche (3) (2014)

	how typical questions in research can be answered by searching through huge text data bases. For example, a platform has been created to make medical abstracts and other academic publications more accessible to researchers. ○ Global Technical Operations is investigating big data technology to optimize biotech production, for example by looking at the incoming data streams. The long-term goal is to develop a system that can help to predict the success or failure of production steps.
Health IT: Interpreting Big Data (Roche Annual Report 2014, p.67, published on 26 January 2015)[76]	• Several initiatives are on-going at Roche to enhance real-world data and real-world evidence capabilities with the aim to make informed decisions on development strategies, improve medical practice and make medicines accessible to the right patient at the right time. • A new function, 'Real World Data Science' (RWD-S), was created in Product Development in 2014. The purpose of RWD-S is to translate RWD into evidence and insights to enable better decisions for medicines to improve patient care. RWD-S serves as a strategic partner with the research, development and commercial organisations and aspires to be an effective connector across the organization.
Ken Wilcox, Head of Pharma Informatics: We Want to Shorten the Research Process (Interview, published on 24 February 2015)[77]	• Roche's IT Centre of Excellence is located in Madrid, Spain and provides support to Big Data projects among other things. • The goal is to shorten the research process and speed up the emergence of medicines while reducing the cost for patients.
Shining Light on Treatment Benefit: How Roche is Leveraging Real World Data to Improve Patient Outcomes (Feature story in Roche media store published on 29 May 2015)[78]	• According to Niko Andre, Head of Global Medical Affairs, Real World Data (RWD), if used appropriately, may be an enormously powerful source of information, providing greater understanding of medicines, diseases and their progression, and the impact of change in treatment standards over time. RWD may also detect new safety signals and explore the real, long-term impact of medicines on patient health.

---

[76] Roche (4) (2015)
[77] Roche (5) (2015)
[78] Roche (6) (2015)

2. Google research

Using the search string '"Roche" AND "big data"' and screening the hits for insights regarding R&D has shown five results of interest:

Source	Insights
Roche follows GSK in move to unlock its data vault on drugs (Article in Fierce Biotech by John Carrol on 26 Feb, 2013)[79]	• Roche will follow GSK's footsteps and will also make its clinical trial data available outside investigators. • Roche will work with an independent group which will be charged with sorting out and approving requests for access to anonymized clinical trial data for all approved products.
Roche, Astra to Share Drug Research Data (Article in The Wall Street Journal by Jeanne Whalen, updated on 25 June 2013)[80]	• Given the risen costs of drug discovery and development, Roche Holding AG and AstraZeneca PLC agreed to share early-stage drug design to try speed up the development of effective medicines. • Under the deal, both companies will contribute data to a third company, MedChemica Ltd. of the U.K., that specializes in scrutinizing chemical compounds to pinpoint structures that tend to create safety or efficacy problems. • By sharing their past design successes and failures, the companies say they hope to increase their odds of building safe and effective drugs.
Big Biological Impacts from Big Data (Article in Science by Mike May, published on 13 June 2014)[81]	• A century's worth of Roche R&D data were more than doubled in 2011–2012 in a single large-scale experiment to sequence hundreds of cancer cell lines. • Scientists at Roche want to derive more value from these data sets and others collected years ago. Thus, they are collaborating with PointCross in Foster City, California, to create a data platform that allows flexible searching of data from the past 25 years of Roche studies, including those outsourced to contract research organizations. Those data, along with information about thousands of compounds, will be mined to use the existing knowledge to develop new drugs.
Roche acquires Bina Technologies and enters the genomic informatics market (Article in PR Newswire, pub-	• Roche announced the acquisition of Bina Technologies, Inc., a privately held company located in California, USA. Bina provides a big data platform for centralized management and processing of next generation se-

---
[79] Carrol (2013)
[80] Whalen (2013)
[81] May (2014)

lished on 19 December 2014)[82]	quencing (NGS) data. • The acquisition by Roche will enable Bina to accelerate product development and global commercialization of the Bina-GMS as an enterprise software system supporting multiple sequencing technologies while developing a solution for Roche sequencing systems. Roche will also continue to grow Bina's unique interdisciplinary team of bioinformatics scientists, computer scientists and software engineers. • Bina will be integrated into Roche Sequencing Unit in Q1 2015 and will continue to focus on expanding its innovative genomic analysis solutions portfolio.
Big Data Helps Find the Achilles Heel of Each Individual Cancer (Post on Nautilus.com by Kat McGowan published on 4 March 2015)[83]	• Roche paid more than a billion dollars to buy about half of a small company called Foundation Medicine. The deal gives Roche access to Foundation's database, which holds the DNA sequences of the tumors of 35,000 cancer patients, along with information about what kinds of drugs they were treated with and how good those drugs were at beating back the cancer. • The deal is part of Roche's efforts in oncology research to develop better-targeted drugs for cancer patients by analyzing DNA sequencing data.

3. Congresses

The screening of websites/abstracts/programs of big data congresses in general or specifically for the pharmaceutical industry has shown six results on Roche and R&D:

Name of congress	Insights
Big Data Events for Pharma (Google search strings: "big data congress pharma"; "big data conference pharma"; "big data summit pharma")	

Oxford Global Annual Pharmaceutical IT Congress
23-24 September 2015
(London, UK)
	• Speakers:
	   o Michael Braxenthaler, Pharma Research and Early Development Informatics, Global Head Strategic Alliances
	   o Juergen Hammer, Global Head Data Science, Center Head Pharma Research and Early Devel-

---

[82] PR Newswire (2014)
[83] McGowan (2015)

	opment Informatics

Oxford Global Pharmaceutical IT World Asia Congress 25-26 March 2014 (Singapore)	• Speakers:
	   o Michael Braxenthaler, Pharma Research and Early Development Informatics, Global Head Strategic Alliances
	   o Juergen Hammer, Global Head Disease and Translational Informatics
	   o Alain Nanzer, Global Area Head Non-Clinical Safety Informatics
	   o Paul Whitehead, pRED Informatics Center Head

Big Data in Clinical Development 2015 7-8 October 2015 (Washington DC, USA)	• **Presentation: Image-based biomarkers to enhance clinical research** *(Dr. Angelika Fuchs, Senor Data Scientist, pRED Informatics)*
Cambridge Healthtech Institute's Seventh Annual Integrated Pharma Informatics & Data Science 16- 18 February 2015 (San Francisco, USA)	• **Presentation: Experience & Challenges of Creating and Implementing a Data Science Function** *(Juergen Hammer, Ph.D., MBA, Roche Pharmaceutical Research and Early Development; Center Head, Informatics/IT; Global Head, Data Science, Roche Innovation Center New York)*
Bio IT World Conference & EXPO 21-23 April 2015 (Boston, USA)	*Workshop: Biologics, Bioassay, and Biospecimen Registration Systems:* • **Presentation: Semantic Backbone for Integrating Biological Registration Systems** *(Martin Romacker, Senior Scientist, Data and Information Architecture, Roche Innovation Center Basel)* • **Presentation: Molecular Registration of Novel and Complex Biologics** *(Rudolf Kinder, Senior Scientist, Roche Innovation Center Penzberg)* • **Presentation: Automated Registration and Visualization of Complex Therapeutic Proteins** *(Clemens Wrzodek, Ph.D., Scientific Software Engineer, Technical Project Manager, Roche Diagnostics GmbH)* • **Presentation: Rapid Integration of Cancer Genomics Data Using Hadoop and Cloudera's Impala** *(Sittichoke Saisanit, Ph.D., Data Scientist, Informatics, Pharmaceutical Research and Early Development Informatics, Roche Innovation Center New York)* *Bioinformatics* • **Presentation: Streamlined Planning, Execution, Da-**

	ta Capture and Analysis of Peptide Preformulation Stability Studies (*Roman Affentranger, Dr. sc. Nat, Head, Small Molecule Discovery Workflows*)

	Software Development
	 • Presentation: Semantic Integration of Unstructured Safety Study Data: Experiences and Outlook (*Alain Nanzer, Ph.D., Global Head Safety & Development Workflows, Pharma Research and Early Development Informatics, Roche Innovation Center Basel*)
	
	 Next-Gen Sequencing Informatics
	 • Presentation: Deep Sequencing Based Analysis of Ig repertoire in Humanized Mice (*Stefan Klostermann, Ph.D., Expert Scientist, Bioinformatics/Data Science, Roche Innovation Center Penzberg*)
	
	 Data Visualization and Exploration Tools
	 • Presentation: Bringing Process, Chemical & Analytical Data Together: Data Mining & Visualization (*Jean-Michel Adam, Ph.D., Senior Principal Scientist, Preclinical CMC Process Research, Roche Pharma Research & Early Development, Roche Innovation Center Basel*)
	
	 • Workshop: The Impact of research informatics on laboratory evolution
	 Instructors:
	   o Javier A. Roa, Global Head of Technical Operations & Research Infrastructure
	   o Mischa J. Huber, Basel Head of Technical Operations & Research Infrastructure
	   o Alexander Rossi, Basel Head Laboratory Information Systems & Support

Cambridge's Healthtech Institute's Biomarker & Diagnostics World Congress 5-7 May 2015 (Philadelphia, USA)	• Presentation: Applying Data Science in Translational Clinical Research (*James Cai, Ph.D., Head, Data Science, Roche*)

5.2.5 Merck & Co

1. Company Website
The research on the company website (www.merck.com) itself showed one result:

Source	Insights
Global Health Innovation – Investment Focus Areas (Webpage in Global Health Innovation section, 2015)[84]	• Merck is investing in Health IT Platforms such as health informatics & analytics to transform Big Data into meaningful information (e.g. Big Data analytics, visualization, post-market informatics) and health data liberation to enable interoperability through aggregation, harmonization and integration (e.g. cloud solutions, privacy and security, data aggregation).

2. Google research
Using the search string ""Merck" AND "big data"" and screening the hits for insights regarding R&D has shown four results of interest:

Source	Insights
Merck Optimizes Manufacturing With Big Data Analytics (Article in InformationWeek by Doug Henschen published on 4 February 2014)[85]	• Success story of optimizing manufacturing of vaccines when Merck IT experts were tasked to use Big Data analytics to understand the reason for higher than usual discard rates on certain vaccines: • IT experts realized quickly that the usual investigative approach involving spreadsheet-based analyses to align all data from disparate systems and spotting abnormalities took months, and storage and memory limits meant researchers could only look at a batch or two at a time. • Built on a Hortonworks Hadoop[86] distribution running on Amazon Web Services, Merck Research Laboratories Data Science Platform turned out to be a better fit for the analysis because Hadoop supports a schema-on-read approach. As a result, data from 16 disparate sources could be used in analysis without having to be transformed with time-consuming and expensive ETL processes to conform to a rigid, predefined relational

---

[84] Merck (2015)
[85] Henschen (2014)
[86] The Hadoop software library is a framework that allows for the distributed processing of large data sets across clusters of computers using simple programming models. It is designed to scale up from single servers to thousands of machines, each offering local computation and storage.

	database schema
	• Through 15 billion calculations and more than 5.5 million batch-to-batch comparisons, Merck discovered that certain characteristics in the fermentation phase of vaccine production were closely tied to yield in a final purification step.
	• As a result, Merck is applying the lessons learnt to various vaccines and will ask regulators to approve the new manufacturing process.
Merck diversifies its Big Data agenda (Article in Medical Marketing & Media by Marc Iskowitz, published on 26 March 2014)[87]	• Merck, through its medical information and innovation unit (M2i2), partners with a list of organizations at the intersection of Big Data and health IT: 　o A partnership with Boston Children's Hospital, announced by M2i2 in late February 2014, seeks to harness publicly available information from Twitter and Facebook to glean insights about insomnia. 　o Along similar lines, M2i2 is also working with the online oncology community Smart Patients. • Furthermore, Merck has announced collaborations with EMR outfits Practice Fusion and Allscripts to co-develop clinical decision support content, as well as with Maccabi Healthcare Services, a two-million-member Israeli healthcare provider, to leverage the provider's longitudinal database and understand how drugs behave in the real world.
Merck Optimizes Critical Drug Development with Revolution Analytics' gsDesign Explorer (Case study in Revolution Analytics, 2015)[88]	• Merck has invested in gsDesign Explorer to collect and analyze massive data sets to complete the clinical trial process in less time resulting into lower costs: 　• "The greatest challenge to pharmaceutical drug development is the large amount of data generated by the sequential testing of experimental therapies. Analyzing these large sets of data can significantly delay a new drug's delivery to patients or just as easily waste resources on drugs that turn out to be inferior to already available standard treatments. GsDesign Explorer significantly reduces the time of data analysis required in sequential drug testing. Recently, we had a trial at Merck that we couldn't have done without gsDesign Explorer. This project allows promising new drugs to

---

[87] Iskowitz (2014)
[88] Revolution Analytics (2015)

Data Governance Initiative created by Hortonworks, Aetna, Merck, Target and SAS (Article in FierceBigData by Pam Baker, published on 2 February 2015)[89]	• Hortonworks, Aetna, Merck, Target and SAS announced the creation of the Data Governance Initiative (DGI) designed to ensure a common approach to data governance across all systems and data. • DGI will also create an audit store, integrate the metadata framework with existing Apache Falcon data life cycle management and Apache Ranger data security projects as well as lay the groundwork for additional long-term initiatives, for example, expose particular data sets via an application programming interface (API) that can be invoked by analytics applications.

3. Congresses

The screening of websites/abstracts/programs of big data congresses in general or specifically for the pharmaceutical industry has shown eleven results on Merck & Co and R&D:

Name of congress	Insights
Big Data Events for Pharma (Google search strings: "big data congress pharma"; "big data conference pharma"; "big data summit pharma")	
Pharma Data Analytics 29 September–1 October 2014 (Brussels, Belgium)	• **Presentation: Exploring Different Methods of Data Mapping: The platform integration challenge for "Going Paperless": an experience report from the veterinarian GxP area** *(Brunhilde Schoelzke, Senior Specialist, R&D Analytics & Data)*

Big Data & Analytics for Pharma Summit
4-5 November 2015
(Philadelphia, USA)
	• Speakers (presentations to be confirmed):
	   o Barnaby Fountain, Director, Business Analytics Realization
	   o Laura Galuchie, Director, Clinical Performance, Analytics & Innovation
	   o Julia O'Neill, Director, Engineering

Big DIP USA 22-24 September 2014 (Boston, USA)	• Sample Speaker: Sachin Jain, Chief Medical Information & Innovation Officer

---

[89] Baker (2015)

Oxford Global Annual Pharmaceutical IT Congress
23-24 September 2015
(London, UK)
	• Speakers:
	   o Jan Hauss, Head Central Analytics Informatics
	   o Dermot McCaul, Director, Preclinical Development and Biologics IT
	   o Andrew Porter, Director, Enterprise Architecture
	   o Martin Ryzl, Director, GIC Analytics Platform Engineering

Oxford Global Pharmaceutical IT World Asia Congress 25-26 March 2014 (Singapore)	• Speakers: o Eike Staub, Computational Biologist
Big Data in Clinical Development 2015 7-8 October 2015 (Washington DC, USA)	• **Presentation: Generating real world evidence and leveraging it to inform clinical trial design, render better decisions and reduce the cost of care** *(Dr. Thomas Tsang, Chief Medical Officer, Merck Healthcare Services and Solution)* • **Panel discussion between heads of clinical development from pharma, biotech and cros** *(Panelist: Roy D. Baynes, MD, PhD, Senior Vice President Global Clinical Development)*
Cambridge Healthtech Institute's Seventh Annual Integrated Pharma Informatics & Data Science 16- 18 February 2015 (San Francisco, USA)	• **Presentation: Enabling Secure Real World Data Exchange and Collaborative Analytics across Healthcare Organizations** *(Patrick Loerch, Director, Health IT, Information Technology)*
Fleming Europe Pharma Exabyte 27-28 May 2015 (Berlin, Germany)	• Speaker: Martin Ryzl, Director, GIC Analytics Platform Engineering
Marcus Evans Annual Pharma Data Analytics 18-19 November 2014 (Philadelphia, USA)	• Speaker: Paul Kallukaran, Executive Director, Global Information Sciences and Analytics: Commercial
Bio IT World Conference & EXPO 21-23 April 2015 (Boston, USA)	• **Workshop:** Biologics, Bioassay, and Biospecimen Registration Systems: o Speaker: Beth Basham, IT Director, Client Services, Biologics & Vaccines Discovery (Talk title to be announced) *Pharmaceutical R&D Informatics* • **Luncheon Presentation II: Where Science Intersects**

	with Business – **Creating Business Dashboards That Combine Data from Multiple Sources** *(Huijun Wang, Ph.D., Associate Principle Scientist, Cheminformatics, Merck & Co (among other speakers from other pharmaceutical/consulting companies)*
	• **Panel discussion: Growing a Data Science Team** *(Moderator: Martin Leach, Ph.D., Vice President,Global Data Office, Biogen; Panelists: Johnson, Ph.D., Associate Vice President, Scientific Informatics, Merck (among other panelists from other pharmaceutical companies)*
	• **Presentation: The Construction of a Scientific Modeling Culture and Technology Platform at Merck** *(Chris L. Waller, Ph.D., Director and Head, Scientific Modeling Platforms, Merck Research Laboratories)*
Real World Evidence & Data Partnerships Summit 14-15 October 2014 (Bethesda, USA)	• **Panel Discussion: Real World Evidence & The Digital Healthcare Space: The Next Frontier?** *(Panelist among other representatives from GSK and Open mHealth: Patirck Howiem Leaderm Customer Data and Applications and General Manager, Comsort)*

5.3 Interpretation and Analysis

The research has shown that all five of the selected pharmaceutical companies are active in Big Data research and are investing in Big Data for their R&D process:

Novartis:

Areas of focus within the R&D process:
Big Data is part of Novartis's mission of dedicating efforts and knowledge to search for treatments and cures for long, healthy lives. Novartis is already using Big Data analytics for drug discovery and clinical trial management in the therapeutic areas of oncology, ophthalmology, and haematology (multiple sclerosis). Moreover, Novartis is investing in Next-Generation Sequencing (NGS).

Resources/infrastructure:
While there are no details available on Novartis' financial investments into Big Data research, it is obvious that the company has made investments in hiring Big Da-

ta scientists and experts in order to re-organize the traditional drug research team and assemble cross-disciplinary teams that also involve data scientists who work closely together with biologists and clinicians to advance drug discovery. Novartis' hub for Big Data research is the Novartis Institute for Biomedical research where experts are currently working on solutions to overcome hurdles such as increasing data size, dimensionality and complexity of data in order to quickly integrate and analyse large volumes of results from pre-clinical and clinical studies and to combine those with available data from external sources to identify potential target molecules. Thereby, Next Generation Sequencing is one of the focus areas at the Institute for Biomedical Research.

In terms of technical infrastructure, Novartis is equipped with a suite of three visualization tools (HTS-Explorer, Chemotography and ConTour) that work synergistically to help researchers visualize data and identify promising drug candidates. Moreover, Novartis has invested in the data system MapR, a technology to integrate diverse data sets from external institutions to accelerate drug research in NGS. The system also facilitates the interactions between computer scientists and life scientists.

Collaboration/Partners:
Novartis' eye care division Alcon has entered into an agreement with Google Inc. to in-license its "smart lens" technology for all ocular medical uses. Alcon has the development and commercialization rights to help diabetic patients manage their disease and people living with presbyopia provide accommodative vision correction. Furthermore, Novartis has agreed on a collaboration with Covance, a drug development service company, to expand the NIBR's existing clinical data warehouse and to develop ways to quickly integrate and analyse large volumes of results from pre-clinical and clinical studies. Moreover, together with Pfizer and Eli Lilly, Novartis has been tasked by the US government with helping to improve ClinicalTrials.gov in order to make it more effective at matching patients to studies. The three pharmaceutical companies are asked to add a machine-readable "target health profile" for 50 clinical trials. Additionally, Novartis announced additional steps to extend its clinical trial data transparency by launching the ideaPoint portal that allows researchers access to patient level data on newly approved innovative medicines in the EU and United States.

Best Practices:
In a collaborative effort with the Necker Children's Hospital-Imagine Foundation, Novartis successfully applied DNA sequencing technologies and analytics to detect the cause of a kidney cancer called glomerulosclerosis.

Pfizer:

Areas of focus within the R&D process:
During the last three years, Pfizer has started making a more conscious choice to use data analytics in more upstream business functions like the R&D and innovation process. Particularly, Pfizer is directing Big Data towards how to tailor treatments for small patient populations while staying highly profitable, how to bring drugs to market faster and thus cutting development costs, and how to develop more efficacious drugs. Pfizer has already been very successful with Big Data analytics for oncology (*Xalkori*), but does also focus its research efforts on fibromyalgia and assesses the value of data in understanding the obesity epidemic and how it may inform medicine development. Moreover, Pfizer is using Big Data analytics for personalized medicine applying biomarker focused research and NGS.

Resources/infrastructure:
At Pfizer the company's Big Data strategy, sits with the Global Data Management (GDM) team. GDM acts as a shared, centralized resource for all functions – mainly for R&D, finance and procurement, commercial, manufacturing and corporate. Since 2013, Pfizer has moved from ETL (extract, transform, load) process to data virtualization tools. In addition to that, Pfizer has established a Precision Medicine Analytics Ecosystem looking for non-obvious patterns between genomic data, clinical trials data and de-identified medical records to draw insights relevant for the future R&D process.
There is no information available on how much budget Pfizer is investing for its Big Data efforts and whether the transformation to a Big Data oriented company has been achieved by hiring external data experts or whether internal staff has been qualified in this area.

Collaboration/partners:
Pfizer has entered a few alliances with companies that are specialized in the field of gathering de-identified data, linking claims data with clinical health records and an-

alyzing data. Pfizer has partnered in the last few years with Humedica, CliniWorks Israel and Optum Labs.

Best Practices:
Pfizer is the only company that has already applied Big Data analytics to successfully launching a new pharmaceutical compound. With the aid of its Precision Medicine Analytics Ecosystem connecting the dots among genomic, clinical trial and anonymous EMR data, Pfizer was able to target a specific patient population that did not respond to available treatment options at that time. In the case of lung cancer, research revealed that about 5% of patients were not engaged in high-risk lifestyles (such as smokers, coal miners or otherwise harm their lungs). However, data analytics showed that they had one thing in common: a mutation in their ALK gene. Pfizer was able to develop Xalkori which was approved in 2011 (at a time when the term Big Data just emerged) specifically for lung cancer patients with the ALK gene.

Sanofi:

Areas of focus within the R&D process:
According to Brian Ellerman, Head of Scouting and Information Science Innovation, harnessing Big Data for R&D is a major priority for Sanofi. However, there is only very little information available in terms of how and for which therapeutic areas Sanofi is using Big Data for drug discovery and clinical trial management. Overall, Sanofi is active in the biomedical disciplines translational medicine and NGS.

Resources/ infrastructure:
There is no information available on how much Sanofi invests from a budget and human resources perspective. Furthermore, no specific technical platforms and tools were mentioned.

Collaboration/partners:
Sanofi has initiated a long-term collaboration with NextBio to incorporate patient omics[90] and clinical data into Sanofi´s drug research and development, as part of

---

[90] The word "omics" indicates the study of a body of information, such as the genome, proteome (study of proteins), metabolism, RNA transcripts and autoantibody profiles.

its Translational Medicines for Patients program. Furthermore, together with Johnson&Johnson, Sanofi is working with IBM Watson to speed up research initiatives, in particular accelerating drug comparative-effectiveness studies. Additionally, Sanofi hopes to speed up its drug-repurposing, which means the discovery of alternative indications for existing drugs. Apart from its partnerships with big data companies, Sanofi has followed GSK to share its clinical trial results on ClinicalStudyDataRequest.com. Moreover, Sanofi has posted three prostate cancer trials on Project Data Sphere, a pharma supported site aimed at using data sharing to speed up the development of new cancer cures. In its efforts to unify procedures followed in clinical trials, Sanofi has helped together with GSK and Roche to found the non-profit organization TransCelerate Bio Pharma to create standards for collecting and reporting clinical trial data. As also stated on its company website, Sanofi believes that making clinical trial data available to the research community promises to advance science and medicine and as such contribute to improvements in public health as well as trust and knowledge about the pharmaceutical drug development.

Best Practices:
There are no concrete examples or success stories available on how Sanofi has leveraged Big Data for its R&D and innovation process.

Roche:

Areas of focus within the R&D process:
According to Roche's company website, several Big Data initiatives, in particular to enhance real-world data (RWD) and real-world evidence (RWE), are ongoing at Roche. Thereby, Roche is very active in the fields of oncology and cancer immunology.

Resources/infrastructure:
A new function, 'Real World Data Science' (RWD-S), was created within the already existing function Product Development in 2014. The purpose of RWD-S is to translate RWD into evidence and insights to enable better decisions to improve patient care. RWD-S serves as a strategic partner for the research, development and commercial organisations and aspires to be an effective connector across the organisations. Moreover, from a pure technology and computer science aspect, Roche has an IT Centre of Excellence, located in Madrid, Spain, that provides

support to Big Data projects among other IT projects at Roche. In addition to that, Roche has established the function Business Intelligence and Master Data Management Informatics that coordinates projects to enhance Big Data technologies at Roche to generate new insights for research projects. Overall, Roche has understood that addressing the Big Data challenge in R&D requires a multidisciplinary approach where biologists, computer scientists, toxicologists, statisticians and chemists have to work in a collaborative way and is focusing its organizational efforts to ensure such an approach is not just theory, but will be put into practice.

In terms of data systems and technologies, it is mentioned that Roche is using Cloudera's Impala[91] and Hadoop for rapid integration and analysis of cancer genomics data.

There is no concrete information available on how much Roche invests from a budget perspective.

Collaboration/Partners:

Aiming to enter the genomic information's market, Roche has acquired Bina Technologies in 2014. Bina provides a Big Data platform for centralized management and processing of NGS data. Bina has been integrated into Roche's Sequencing Unit in Q1 2015 to develop innovative genomic analysis solutions for Roche. Furthermore, Roche has paid more than a billion dollars to buy about half of a small company, called Foundation Medicine. The deal gives Roche access to Foundation's database, which holds the DNA sequences of the tumors of 35,000 cancer patients along with therapies and drug response information. Moreover, Roche and AstraZeneca agreed to share early-stage drug research data aiming to speed up the development of effective medicines by cutting down drug discovery costs. Under the deal, both companies will contribute data to a third company, MedChemica that specializes in scrutinizing chemical compounds to pinpoint structures that tend to create safety or efficacy problems.

Adding to the aspect of data transparency, Roche will also follow GSK and other pharmaceutical companies to make its clinical trial data available outside investigators. Thereby, Roche will work with an independent group, which will be charged with sorting out, and approving requests for access to anonymized clinical trial data for all approved products.

---

[91] Cloudera Impala is Cloudera's open source massively parallel processing (MPP) SQL (structured query language) query engine for data stored in a computer cluster running Apache Hadoop.

Best Practices:
While Roche has started to build up the infrastructure and initiated collaborations to gain access to external data pools, the company is still in the early stages and has at least not publically shared a Big Data success story that could be regarded as a best practice case study by others.

Merck & Co:

Areas of focus within the R&D process:
Merck is investing in health IT and data platforms in the therapeutic areas of oncology, vaccines, insomnia and animal health.

Resources/infrastructure:
Merck has integrated a function called medical information and innovation unit (M2i2) that has initiated partnerships with a couple of organizations at the intersection of Big Data and Health IT. Other than that, there is no information available on the responsibilities of this department and how Merck is set up for Big Data initiatives and projects in general – neither from a budget nor from a human resources perspective. In terms of data technologies, Merck has invested in gsDesign Explorer to collect and analyze massive data aiming to complete the clinical trial process in less time resulting in lower costs. Furthermore, Merck is using Hortonworks Hadoop software that allows analyzing data from disparate sources.

Collaboration/Partners:
Through its M2i2 unit, Merck has partnered with a list of organizations such as the Boston Children's Hospital in 2014. The partnership seeks to harness publicly available information from Twitter and Facebook to glean insights about insomnia. Along similar lines, M2i2 is also working with the oncology community Smart Patients. Moreover, Merck has announced collaborations with EMR outfits Practice Fusion and Allscripts to co-develop clinical decision support content, as well as with Maccabi Healthcare Services, to leverage the provider's longitudinal database to understand how drugs operate in the real world.

Merck has also partnered with Hortonworks, Aetna, Target and SAS for the creation of the Data Governance Inititative (DGI) designed to ensure a common approach to data governance across all systems and data. Moreover, Merck has partnered with Elsevier to develop a series of dashboards that can combine information from multiple sources to create views with facets for drug, target and disease related information.

Best Practices:

Merck IT experts have successfully used Big Data technologies to find the reason for higher than usual discard rates on certain vaccines. IT experts realized quickly that the usual investigative approach involving spreadsheet-based analyses to align all data from disparate systems and spotting abnormalities would take months. Additionally, storage and memory limits meant researchers could only look at a batch or two at a time. Built on Hortonworks Hadoop distribution software that ran on Amazon Web Service, Merck's research laboratories Data Science Platform turned out to be a better fit for the analysis since Hadoop supports a schema-on-read approach which means that data from 16 disparate sources could be used in one analysis without having to be transformed with time-consuming and expensive ETL processes. Finally, through 15 billion calculations and more than 5.5 million batch-to-batch comparisons, Merck discovered that certain characteristics in the fermentation phase of the vaccine production were closely tied to the yield in a final purification step. As a result, Merck now applies the lessons learnt to various vaccines and will ask regulators to approve the new manufacturing process.

6. Conclusion: Derived strategies to leverage Big Data for R&D

As a conclusion, all five companies are looking into ways to use Big Data for drug discovery and clinical trial management. Thereby, oncology and the associated field of next generation sequencing are the areas of highest interest. Moreover, all companies have partnered with external companies that are either specialized in Big Data technologies or have access to additional data sources. The transparency of clinical data is also for the majority of the examined companies an important topic. While the trend to make clinical data available to the public has been primarily driven by the public mistrust in clinical trials sponsored by pharmaceutical companies, a positive benefit is that it also enhances data sharing across companies, academics and researchers. Overall, the research has demonstrated that Big Pharma has committed its research efforts on Big Data for R&D and the innovation process. However, Big Data research is still in its early stages looking at the only very few case studies available to date.

The following conclusions have been drawn based on publically available sources and information, which implicates limitations concerning the level of detail and accuracy of the research findings:

	Big Data for R&D	Therapeutic/ Research Areas	Alliances/ Partners	Clinical trial data transparency	Data technology infrastructure	Best Practice Case Study
NOVARTIS	✓	• Oncology • Ophthalmology • Haematology (Multiple Sclerosis) • NGS	• Google • Covance	✓	• MapR • HTS Explorer • Chemotopgraphy • ConTour	• Detection of glomerulo-sclerosis as cause of kidney cancer
Pfizer	✓	• Oncology • Fibromyalgia • Obesity • Biomarker-focused research • Personalized medicine • NGS	• Humedica • CliniWorks • Optum Labs	✗	• Precision Medicine Analytics Ecosystem	• Xalkori
SANOFI	✓	• NGS • Translational medicine	• NextBio • IBM Watson	✓		✗
Roche	✓	• Oncology • NGS • RWD/RWE	• Bina Technologies • Foundation Medicine • Astra Zeneca • Point Cross	✓	• Cloudera Impala • Hadoop	✗
MERCK	✓	• Oncology • Vaccines • Animal Health	• Smart Patients • Practice Fusion • Allscripts • DGI	✗	• GsDesign Explorer • Hadoop	• Optimization of manufacturing of vaccines

Figure 13: Summary of the results of the online research
Source: Own illustration

6.1 Infrastructure

In order to implement a Big Data infrastructure to fully explore the existent and prospective capabilities of Big Data for the R&D process, pharmaceutical companies should focus on the following three pillars:

1. Data

Pharmaceutical companies have to ensure they have access and the right technologies at hand in order to gather, collect and store data. Therefore, they should focus their efforts on the following dimensions of data quality:

The 7 dimensions of data quality

Dimensions	Characteristics
Accuracy	Data precisely reflects the objective or transaction it describes
Reliability	Data is consistent across multiple transactions
Credibility	The degree to which decision makers trust both the accuracy and reliability of data
Timeliness	Data is available to the information consumer when it is needed
Appropriateness	The degree to which the data itself is relevant to the needs of an organization
Completeness	All of the relevant or required data is readily available for use when required

Figure 14: The 7 dimensions of data quality
Source: Morabito (2015), p.98

2. Analytics Tools
Data alone do not provide the insights to leverage the R&D process. It is important that companies invest into analytic tools to bring the different data sources together and to correlate and analyze them in order to derive new and relevant insights out of the large amounts of data (see appendix 5 and 6 for the architecture and established Big Data analytics tools).

3. Expertise
A Big Data infrastructure does also require the right skill sets and a suitable and sufficiently trained workforce. Pharmaceutical companies will probably have to complement their research teams with a new profession: the data scientist. It is crucial that companies implement a multi-disciplinary approach where biologists, computer scientists, toxicologists, statisticians, chemists and data scientists work in a collaborative way in order to make the most value out of the gathered data and the applied analytic tools.

Furthermore, companies should also consider establishing an overseeing function to coordinate the big data projects from their beginning within the organization, ensure alignment across multiple functions and control that Big Data initiatives are in line with the industry's policies and privacy rules, but also have an eye on competitor's activities in the field of Big Data and ensure constant learning of the organization as new knowledge about Big Data techniques and best practices will continuously become available.

6.2 Interoperability

Strategies to increase interoperability regarding health data can foster Big Data for R&D in many ways. As described in chapter 4.3, the different stakeholders within the healthcare sector such as providers, payors, pharmaceutical companies and academia own different types of data. While one of the major reasons for these data silos is the privacy law protecting the individual's health data, there is still the opportunity to partner with, for example universities or hospitals on a project level, to expand the company's available data for specific research purposes if patients provide informed consent. The online research has demonstrated that this kind of partnership is feasible and has shown first success to leverage Big Data for clinical trial programs. The trend of clinical trial data transparency does also have the positive 'side effect' that pharmaceutical companies and other stakeholders have access to external clinical trial data in order to avoid duplication of clinical trials and foster innovation.

Moreover, pharmaceutical companies should also think about acquisitions and collaborations with Big Data technology companies to get access to advanced dashboards, data technologies and experienced data scientists to advance the company's own Big Data expertise.

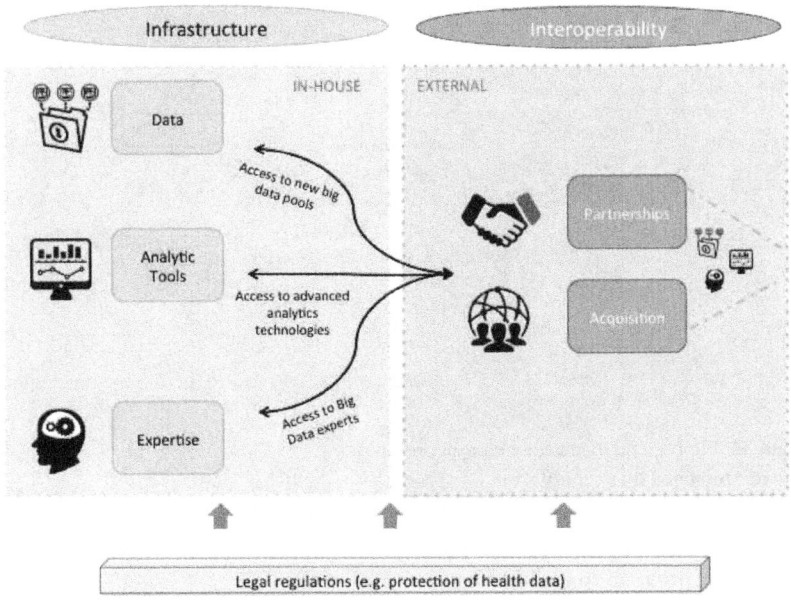

Figure 15: The Big Data framework for pharmaceutical companies
Source: Own illustration

6.3 Big Data Business Intelligence

Big Data should not just be treated as the isolated 'guinea pig' in the company's research labs. In order to fully explore the existent and prospective capabilities of Big Data, organizations should fully embed Big Data into their business models. This allows pooling and sharing of derived insights across all units within the organization along the innovation process and life cycle of a pharmaceutical compound. Moreover, the buy-in of the senior management usually enables a proper build-up of a consistent infrastructure dedicating more efforts and budget towards Big Data initiatives.

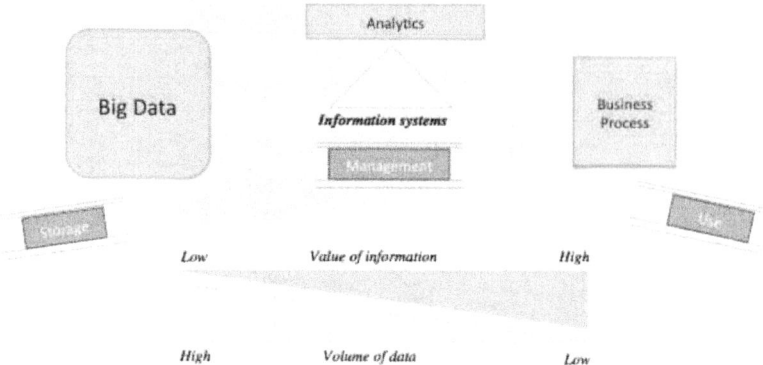

Figure 16: Big Data management within an organization
Source: Morabito (2015), p.179

Therefore, it is important for companies to expand the scope of their existing data governance program to include big data.

> Data Governance is defined as a system of decision rights and accountabilities for information-related processes, executed according to agreed-upon models which describe who can take what actions with what information, and when, under what circumstances, using what methods (Data Governance Institute (DGI), 2015)[92].

> According to Soares (2013) Big data governance is part of a broader information governance program that formulates policy relating to the optimization, privacy, and monetization of big data by aligning the objectives of multiple functions. [93]

---

[92] The Data Governance Institute (2015), p.3
[93] Soares (2013), p.4

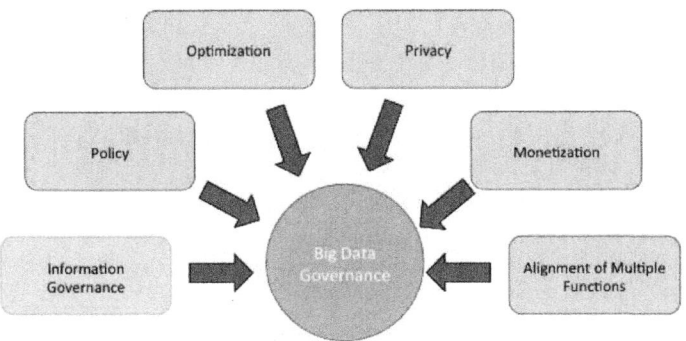

Figure 17: Overview of key components of Big Data Governance
Source: Morabito (2015), p.87

Another pre-requisite is that the Big Data strategy of a company is in line with the overall corporate strategy. Only when the organization has a clear picture about what it wants to achieve, it can determine which business processes and areas of Big Data can and should be of use. For example, if a pharmaceutical company is striving towards becoming a leader in personalized medicine, Big Data has the claimed potential to open new doors in this area of research identifying niche patient populations and designing better-targeted drugs. In order to guarantee coordination and consistency of Big Data systems and processes, organizations need to establish a central function that manages Big Data across departments. The overall scope of this function is to ensure clarity on various aspects of data access, integration, usage, management and ownership of Big Data management[94]. Big Data Governance is also closely linked to the identification of the required infrastructure for a specific Big Data project, which represents a fundamental part of the Big Data capabilities of a company. Only the best suitable data technologies and analytics tools as well expertise set the course for advances in Big Data research and success within the organization.

---

[94] Morabito (2015), p.101

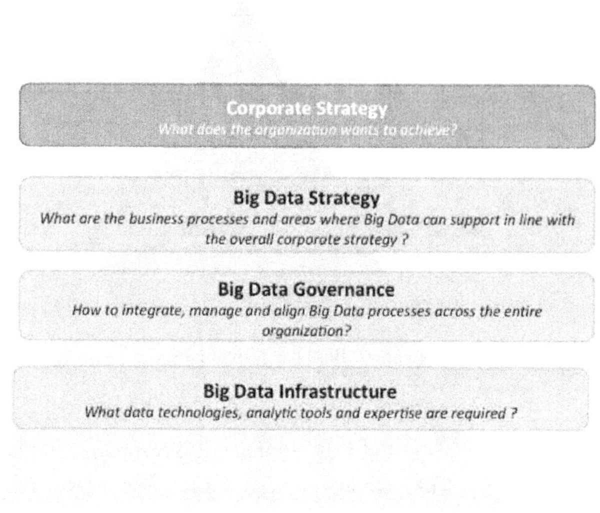

Corporate Strategy
What does the organization wants to achieve?

Big Data Strategy
What are the business processes and areas where Big Data can support in line with the overall corporate strategy?

Big Data Governance
How to integrate, manage and align Big Data processes across the entire organization?

Big Data Infrastructure
What data technologies, analytic tools and expertise are required?

Figure 18: Process of implementing Big Data in alignment with the overall corporate strategy
Source: Adapted from Morabito (2015), p.88

7. Key findings and future outlook

Streamlining the R&D process is of great interest for Big Pharma given the high costs that have exploded over the last two decades as well as the stricter regulation standards of the health authorities worldwide. Big Data has a claimed potential to accelerate the innovation process and allowing research in niche areas for more targeted and individualized therapy options. The online research has demonstrated that all of the top five pharmaceutical companies have started to integrate Big Data into their R&D process. Novartis for example is even promoting Big Data as part of their innovative research approach in order to fulfil their company's mission of "cures for long healthy lifes". Although there is no concrete data publically available on the overall investment that has been allocated in terms of budget and human resources, the conclusion can be drawn from the online research data that there have been investments, irrespective of the concrete amount, in data and analytics technologies as well as collaborations with different external institutions such as academia, healthcare service provider and global IT players (e.g. Google and IBM Watson) or even acquisitions of other Big Data technology companies. However, there are differences between the five companies in terms of the level of implementation and overall integration of Big Data in the organization and across functions. Roche and Pfizer have already implemented a centralized function that manages, aligns and further establishes Big Data within the organization. At other companies Big Data is only rolled out in the research hubs (e.g. Novartis Institute for Biomedical Research) as pilots to better understand how the data phenomenon can be best applied for the innovation process. Thereby, the number one research area of Big Data for the companies, which were in focus of this online research, is oncology.

As of now, there has been just one successful example of Big Data application within the innovation process that has demonstrated that it helps to shape clinical trial design and outcomes: the development of Xalkori by Pfizer for a specific population of lung cancer patients that is lacking the ALK gene. Apart from that example, there have been only smaller benefits observed such as the optimization of manufacturing of vaccines as an example for Merck or Novartis' detection of glomerulosclerosis as a cause of kidney cancer. Hence, these first results prove that Big Data is a promising research field. Nevertheless, it is too early to draw a definite conclusion that Big Data does have an accelerating effect for R&D as it has not yet demonstrated a significance difference in either the duration of research, increase in the probability that a drug surpasses all phases of drug development and clinical trials or reduction of cost. However, it is important to bear in mind that Big Pharma has just started to embrace Big Data and is still in the early stages of learning how to deal with the overwhelming amounts of unstructured data and how to integrate it and correlate it with the data it has already generated. Furthermore, analytics tools have just evolved and only academic scholars have started to extract value out of the massive data pools and bring them into perspective for concrete business and research needs. For most industry leaders, the real potential of Big Data is still a question mark and as the development of a drug takes on average 14 years it will probably take another decade of combined research in Big Data and drug development until there will be an answer available.

8. Reference List

- AmazonWebServices, 2015. *AWS Case Study: Novartis* (Online). Available at: https://aws.amazon.com/de/solutions/case-studies/novartis/. Last accessed September 2015.

- Baker, P., 2015. Data Governance Initiative created by Hortonworks, Aetna, Merck, Target and SAS. *FierceBigData* (online), 2 February 2015. Available at: http://www.fiercebigdata.com/story/data-governance-initiative-created-hortonworks-aetna-merck-target-and-sas/2015-02-02. Last accessed February 2015.

- Baghudana, A., 2015. Pfizer: From Data-Supported to Date-Enabled. *Open Forum* (online), 14 April 2015. Available at: https://openforum.hbs.org/challenge/understand-digital-transformation-of-business/data/pfizer-from-data-supported-to-data-enabled. Last accessed September 2015.

- Carrol, J., 2013. Roche follows GSK in move to unlock its data vault on drugs. *Fierce Biotech* (online), 26 February 2013. Available at: http://www.fiercebiotech.com/story/roche-follows-gsk-move-unlock-its-data-vault-drugs/2013-02-26. Last accessed September 2015.

- Cattell J., Chilukuri, S., Levy, M., 2013. How Big Data can revolutionize pharmaceutical R&D. *Mc Kinsey & Company (online)*, April 2013. Available at: http://www.mckinsey.com/insights/health_systems_and_services/how_big_data_can_revolutionize_pharmaceutical_r_and_d. Last accessed 8 April 2015.

- Citeline, 2015. *Pharma R&D Annual Review 2015* (Online). Available at: https://citeline.com/wpcontent/uploads/RDAnnulReviewReport_Infographic_2015.pdf. Last accessed September 2015.

- ClinDev.Eu, 2013. *Sanofi partners with 'Big Data' firm to enhance translational medicine* (Online), 1 May 2013. Available at: http://www.clindev.eu/sanofi-partners-with-big-data-firm-to-enhance-translational-medicine/. Last accessed May 2015.

- Council of the European Union, 2014. *Proposal for a Regulation of the European Parliament and of the Council on the protection of individuals with regard to the processing of personal data and on the free movement of such data* (General Data Protection Regulation), (Online). Available at: http://www.eudataprotectionlaw.com/wp-content/uploads/2015/01/Regulation-Council-Draft-Dec14.pdf. Last accessed July 2015.

- Datanami, 2015. *Creating Flexible Big Data Solutions for Drug Discovery*, (Online). Available at: http://www.datanami.com/2015/01/19/creating-flexible-big-data-solutions-drug-discovery/. Last accessed 1 May 2015.

- Demos Europe, 2014. *Big & open data in Europe: A growth engine or a missed opportunity?* (Online). Available at: http://www.bigopendata.eu/full-report/. Last accessed: December 2014.

- Ding, M., Eliashberg, J., Stremersch, S., 2014. *Innovation and Marketing in the Pharmaceutical Industry.* 1sted. New York: Springer.

- European Commission (1), 2013. *EU R&D Scoreboard,* (Online). Available at: http://iri.jrc.ec.europa.eu/scoreboard13.html. Last accessed June 2015.

- European Commission (2), 2013. *The economic and social benefits of big data.* SPEECH/13/450, (Online). Available at: http://europa.eu/rapid/press-release_SPEECH-13-450_en.htm. Last accessed August 2014.

- European Commission, 2014. *Towards a thriving data-driven economy*, (Online). Available at: https://ec.europa.eu/digital-agenda/en/news/communication-data-driven-economy. Last accessed July 2015.

- European Convention, 2000. *EU Charter on fundamental human rights.* (Online) Available at: http://www.europarl.europa.eu/charter/pdf/text_en.pdf. Last accessed July 2015.

- European Parliament, 1995. *Directive 95/46/EC of the European Parliament and of the Council of 24 October 1995 on the protection of individuals with regard to the processing of personal data on the free movement of such data,* (Online). Available at: http://eur-lex.europa.eu/LexUriServ/LexUriServ.do?uri=CELEX:31995L0046:en:HTML. Last accessed July 2015.

- Eurosocap, x. *European Standards on Confidentiality and Privacy in Healthcare* (online). Available at: https://www.google.de/url?sa=t&rct=j&q=&esrc=s&source=web&cd=1&ved=0ahUKEwjF7YuV597KAhWLkywKHTpoDZoQFgghMAA&url=https%3A%2F%2Fwww.dataprotection.ie%2Fdocuments%2Fconferences%2FMcClelland.ppt&usg=AFQjCNFNpxi8Yw1kTfAISE664a9uC7K8Hg. Last accessed September 2015.

- Garde, D., 2014. Covance and Novartis team up with eyes on Big Data. *FierceCRO*, (online) 13 October 2014. Available at: http://www.fiercecro.com/story/covance-and-novartis-team-eyes-big-data/2014-10-13. Last accessed May 2015.

- Gartner IT Glossary, 2013. *Big Data*, (Online). Available at: http://www.gartner.com/it-glossary/big-data. Last accessed 8 May 2015.

- Gassmann, O. et al, 2008. *Leading Pharmaceutical Innovation, Trends and Drivers for Growth in the Pharmaceutical Industry.* 2nd ed. Heidelberg: Springer

- Gassmann, O., Reepmeyer, G., Von Zedtwitz, M., 2015. *Leading Pharmaceutical Innovation.* 2nd ed. Heidelberg: Springer.

- Germano, G., 2015. How Pfizer Is Using Big Data To Power Patient Care. *Forbes* (online), 17 February 2015. Available at: http://www.forbes.com/sites/matthewherper/2015/02/17/how-pfizer-is-using-big-data-to-power-patient-care/. Last accessed 3 May 2015.

- Henschen, D., 2014. Merck Optimizes Manufacturing With Big Data Analytics. *Information Week* (online), 4 February 2014. Available at: http://www.informationweek.com/strategic-cio/executive-insights-and-inno-

- vation/merck-optimizes-manufacturing-with-big-data-analytics/d/d-id/1127901. Last accessed September 2015.

- Henschen, D., 2014. Pfizer Connects Dots To Deliver Better Treatments. *InformationWeek* (online), 2 April 2014. Available at: http://www.informationweek.com/strategic-cio/executive-insights-and-innovation/pfizer-connects-dots-to-deliver-better-treatments/d/d-id/1141527. Last accessed May 2015.

- Hordern, V., 2015. Will the New EU Data Protection Regulation Facilitate Healthcare Innovation. *E-Health Law and Policy* (Online), 26 January 2015. Available at: http://www.hldataprotection.com/2015/01/articles/international-eu-privacy/will-eu-data-protection-regulation-facilitate-healthcare-innovation/. Last accessed July 2015.

- Iafrate, F., 2015. *From Big Data to Smart Data.* 1st ed. London: Iste

- IMS Health, 2012. *Big data: Raising the table stakes for master data management*, (Online). Available at: https://www.imshealth.com/deployedfiles/imshealth/Global/Content/Services/Information%20Management/Master%20Data%20Management/Big%20Data%20ebook_FINAL.pdf. Last accessed June 2015.

- iNFORMATICA, 2013. *Big Data for the Pharmaceutical Industry*, (online). Available at: https://www.informatica.com/content/dam/informatica-com/global/amer/us/collateral/executive-brief/big-data-pharmaceutical-industry_ebook_234 1.pdf. Last accessed 12 April 2015.

- International Organization of Standardization, 2015. *ISO/IEC 2382:2015: Information technology- Vocabulary- Part 1: Fundamental terms*, (Online). Available at: https://www.iso.org/obp/ui/#iso:std:iso-iec:2382:ed-1:v1:en. Last accessed July 2015.

- Iskowitz, M., 2014. Merck diversifies its Big Data agenda. *Medical Marketing* (online), 26 March 2014. Available at: http://www.mmm-online.com/channel/merck-diversifies-its-big-data-agenda/article/338259/. Last accessed September 2015.

- James, J., 2012. *How Much Data is Created every Minute?* Domo (online), 8 June 2012. Available at: https://www.domo.com/blog/2012/06/how-much-data-is-created-every-minute/. Last accessed September 2015.

- Landow, Y., 2013. The patient Big Data challenge: Big Data & Analytics for Pharma conference. *Treato Blog* (online), 18 June 2013. Available at: http://blog.treato.com/the-patient-big-data-challenge-big-data-analytics-for-pharma-conference/. Last accessed September 2015.

- Laskowski N., 2013. Pfizer swaps out ETL for data virtualization tools. *TechTaregt.com* (online), February 2013. Available at: http://searchdatamanagement.techtarget.com/feature/Pfizer-swaps-out-ETL-for-data-virtualization-tools. Last accessed May 2015.

- Luchette, M., 2014. Broad and Novartis Keep Up with Big Data. *Bio IT World*, (Online) 15 May 2014. Available at: http://www.bio-itworld.com/2014/5/15/broad-novartis-keep-up-big-data.html. Last accessed May 2015.

- Manyika, J. et al., 2011. Big data: The next frontier for innovation, competition, and productivity. *McKinsey &Company* (online), June 2011. Available at: http://www.mckinsey.com/insights/business_technology/big_data_the_next_frontier_for_innovation. Last accessed September 2015.

- MapR Technologies, 2015. *Novartis Relies on MapR for Flexible Big Data Solutions for Drug Discovery* (Online). Available at: https://www.mapr.com/resources/novartis-relies-mapr-flexible-big-data-solutions-drug-discovery. Last accessed September 2015.

- May, M., 2014. Big biological Impacts from Big Data. *Science* (online), 13 June 2014. Available at: http://www.sciencemag.org/site/products/lst_20140613.xhtml. Last accessed September 2015.

- McAllister, G., 2011. Drug Discovery in the Era of Big Data. *Novartis*, (Online), 19 January 2015. Available at: http://www.conf.slac.stanford.edu/xldb11/talks/xldb2011_wed_1100_Novartis.pdf. Last accessed 28 April 2015.

- McGowan, K., 2015. Big Data Helps Find the Achilles Heel of Each Individual Cancer. *Nautilus.com* (online), 4 March 2015. Available at: http://m.nautil.us/blog/big-data-helps-find-the-achilles-heel-of-each-individual-cancer. Last accessed September 2015.

- Merck, 2015. *Global Health Innovation – Investment Focus Areas* (online). Available at: http://www.merck.com/ghi/focus_areas.html. Last accessed September 2015.

- Morabito, V., 2015. *Big Data and Analytics*. 1st ed. Cham: Springer.

- Morgon, PA., 2015. *Sustainable Development for the Healthcare Industry. Sustainable Development for the Healthcare Industry*. 1st edition. Heidelberg: Springer International Publishing.

- Novartis, 2014. *Novartis extends leadership in clinical trial data transparency, reinforcing its support of clinical research and innovation* (online), 26 February 2014. Available at: https://www.novartis.com/news/media-releases/novartis-extends-leadership-clinical-trial-data-transparency-reinforcing-its. Last accessed September 2015.

- Novartis, 2015. *A normal life is extraordinary* (Online), 19 May 2015. Available at: https://www.novartis.com/stories/hope/normal-life-extraordinary. Last accessed July 2015.

- O´Brien, T., 2013. *Surfing the Wave of Big Data Analytics*. Novartis (online), 27 Oct 2014. Available at:

http://www.novartis.com/stories/discovery/2013-10-big-data.shtml. Last accessed September 2015.

- Petri, T., 2015. *Datenflut und Datenschutz* presented at: Jahrestagung Deutscher Ethikrat "Die Vermessung des Menschen – Big Data und Gesundheit, (Online) 21. Mai 2015. Available at: http://www.ethikrat.org/veranstaltungen/jahrestagungen/die-vermessung-des-menschen. Last accessed July 2015.

- Petrova, E., 2014. Innovation in the Pharmaceutical Industry: *The Process of Drug Discovery and Development. In:* Ding, M., Eliashberg, J., Stremersch, S., ed. 2014. *Innovation and Marketing in the Pharmaceutical Industry*, New York: Springer. *Ch 2*.

- Pfizer, 2012. *Humedica and Pfizer Form Strategic Alliance* (Online), 20 December 2012. Available at: http://www.pfizer.com/sites/default/files/partnering/recent_partnership/122012_humedica_press_release_2.pdf. Last accessed May 2015.

- Pfizer, 2013. *Pfizer US Medical, Scientific, Patent and Civic Organization Funding Report Q3 2013* (Online), 26 November 2013. Available at: http://www.pfizer.com/files/responsibility/grants_contributions/pfizer_us_grants_cc_q4_2013.pdf. Last accessed September 2015.

- Pfizer, 2014. *CliniWorks Forms a Strategic Alliance with Pfizer to Develop a Population Health Management Platform with Advanced Analytics and Patient Care Capabilities* (Online), 7 July 2014. Available at: http://www.pfizer.com/news/press-release /press-release-detail/cliniworks_ forms_a_strategic_alliance_with_pfizer_to_develop_a_population_health_management_platform_with_advanced _analytics_and_patient_care_capabilities. Last accessed May 2015.

- Phacilitate.co.uk, 2014. *Interview with Brian Ellerman* (Online). Available at: http://www.phacilitate.co.uk/news/interview-with-brian-ellerman/. Last accessed May 2015.

- PR newswire, 2014. *Roche acquires Bina Technologies and enters the genomic informatics market* (online), 19 December 2014. Available at: http://www.prnewswire.com/search-results/news/roche%2520and%2520big%2520data-30-days-page-1-pagesize-20. Last accessed September 2015.

- Process Excellence Network, 2014. *6 Ways Pharmaceutical Companies are Using Big Data to Drive Innovation & Value*, (Online). Available at: http://www.bigdatainpharma.com/redForms.aspx?eventid=1000245&id=389080&FormID=11&frmType=1&m=29322&FrmBypass=False&mLoc=F&SpnsorOpt=False. Last accessed 8 April 2015.

- Purdue University, 2012. *Challenges and Opportunities with Big Data*, (Online). Available at: http://www.purdue.edu/discoverypark/cyber/assets/pdfs/BigDataWhitePaper.pdf. Last accessed July 2015.

- PwC, 2012. *From vision to decision. Pharma 2020*, (Online). Available at: http://www.pwc.com/gx/en/pharma-life-sciences/pharma2020/vision-to-decision.jhtml. Last accessed 7 June 2015.

- Raghupathi W, Raghupathi V., 2014. *Big data analytics in healthcare: promise and potential*. Health Information Science and Systems. 2014: 2-3.

- Revolution Analytics, 2015. *Merck optimizes Critical Drug Development with Revolution Analytics´ gsDesign Explorer* (online). Available at: http://www.revolutionanalytics.com/content/merck-optimizes-clinical-drug-development-revolution-analytics-gsdesign-explorer. Last accessed September 2015.

- Roche (1), 2014. *Extracting value from the data deluge* (Online), 28 February 2014. Available at: http://www.roche.com/media/store/roche_stories/roche-stories-2014-01-22.htm. Last accessed September 2015.

- Roche (2). *Big Data* (Online), 10 June 2014. Available at: http://www.roche.com/research_and_development/what_we_are_working_o

n/research_technologies/informatics-based_technologies/big_data.htm. Last accessed September 2015.

- Roche (3), 2014. *Big Data – Revealing the unseen* (Online), 21 July 2014. Available at:
http://www.roche.com/media/store/roche_stories/roche-stories-2014-07-21.htm. Last accessed September 2015.

- Roche (4), 2015. *Health IT: Interpreting Big Data* (Online). *In:* Roche, 2015. *Roche Annual Report 2014*, 26 January 2015, *p.67*. Available at:
http://www.roche.com/gb14e.pdf. Last accessed September 2015.

- Roche (5), 2015. *Ken Wilcox, Head of Pharma Informatics We want to shorten the research process* (Online), 24 February 2015. Available at:
http://www.roche.com/es/careers/spain/service/ken_wilcox_head_of1.htm. Last accessed September 2015.

- Roche (6), 2015. *Shining light on treatment benefit: How Roche is leveraging Real World Data to improve patient outcomes* (Online), 29 May 2015. Available at:
http://www.roche.com/media/store/roche_stories/asco-2015-overview/asco-2015-story-3.htm. Last accessed September 2015.

- Sanofi, 2015. *Clinical trials: Our Data Sharing Commitments* (Online). Available at:
http://en.sanofi.com/rd/clinical_trials/our_data_sharing_commitments/our_data_sharing_commitments.aspx. Last accessed September 2015.

- Schätti, G. and Thier, J., 2014. Big Pharma heiratet Big Data. *Blick*, (Online) 16 July, 2014. Available at:
http://www.blick.ch/news/wirtschaft/big-pharma-heiratet-big-data-was-haben-novartis-und-google-vor-id2987856.html. Last accessed 9 May 2015.

- Schuhmacher, A., 2015. Can Innovation Still Be the Main Growth Driver of the Pharmaceutical Industry? In: Morgon, PA, ed. 2015. *Sustainable Development for the Healthcare Industry*, Heidelberg: Springer International Publishing. Ch 2.

- Silverman, E., 2014. Sanofi Will Share Clinical trial Data, But There Is A Caveat. *Forbes* (online), 2 January 2014. Available at: http://www.forbes.com/sites/edsilverman/2014/01/02/sanofi-will-share-clinical-trial-data-but-there-is-a-caveat/. Last accessed 3 May 2015.

- Soares, S., 2012. *Big Data Governance: An Emerging Imperative*. 1st ed., Boise: MC PressOnline.

- Sommerfeldt, N. and Zschäpitz, H., 2014. *Der Mann, der den Krebs mit viel Geld besiegen will.* Die Welt (online), 24 April 2014. Available at: http://www.welt.de/wirtschaft/article127241953/Der-Mann-der-den-Krebs-mit-viel-Geld-besiegen-will.html. Last accessed September 2015.

- Statista, 2015. *Top 20 global pharmaceutical companies based on pharma revenue in 2014* (in million U.S. dollars), (Online). Available at: http://www.statista.com/statistics/281306/major-global-pharmaceutical-companies-based-on-pharma-revenue-2012/. Last accessed May 2015.

- Taylor, NP., 2013. *Lilly, Novartis and Pfizer sign up to improve ClinicalTrials.gov*. Fierce Biotech IT (online), 24 November 2013. Available at: http://www.fiercebiotechit.com/story/lilly-novartis-and-pfizer-sign-improve-clinicaltrialsgov/2013-11-24. Last accessed September 2015.

- The Data Governance Institute, 2015. *Definitions of Data Governance* (online). Available at: http://www.datagovernance.com/adg_data_governance_definition/. Last accessed September 2015.

- Thomason Reuters, 2015. *Big Data and the needs of the pharma industry* (online), 13 July 2013. Available at: http://ip-science.thomsonreuters.com/info/bigdata/. Last accessed 14 April 2015.

- Twachtman, G., 2014. Pfizer Seeks Insights Into Big Data Analysis, Personalized Medicine Through Optum Labs. *The Pink Sheet* (online) 24 February 2014. Available at:

https://www.optum.com/content/dam/optum/resources/articles/Optum-Labs-Pink-Sheet-04-24-2014.pdf. Last accessed 4 May 2015.

- Weintraub, A., 2014. Big Pharma Opens Up Its big Data. *MIT Technology Review* (online), 21 July 2014. Available at: http://www.technologyreview.com/news/529046/big-pharma-opens-up-its-big-data/. Last accessed May 2015.

- Whalen, J., 2013. Roche, Astra to Share Drug Research Data. *The Wall Street Journal* (online), 25 June 2013. Available at: http://www.wsj.com/articles/SB10001424127887323998604578567682985587790. Last accessed September 2015.

9. Appendices

Appendix 1: Top 10 Pharma Companies by Size of Pipeline.........................95
Appendix 2: List of Big Data congresses...96
Appendix 3: Detailed results - online research on presence at congresses.........101
Appendix 4: Conceptual Architecture of Big Data Analytics.......................122
Appendix 5: Platforms & tools for Big Data analytics in healthcare................124

Appendix 1: Top 10 Pharma Companies by Size of Pipeline

POSITION 2015 (2014)	COMPANY	NO OF DRUGS IN PIPELINE 2015 (2014)	NO OF ORIGINATED DRUGS 2015
1 (1)	GlaxoSmithKline	258 (261)	163
2 (3)	Novartis	245 (223)	182
3 (2)	Roche	234 (248)	158
4 (5)	AstraZeneca	222 (197)	121
5 (8)	Johnson & Johnson	204 (164)	100
6 (6)	Merck & Co	199 (186)	130
7 (4)	Pfizer	199 (205)	132
8 (7)	Sanofi	184 (180)	84
9 (10)	Takeda	130 (132)	68
10 (11)	Eli Lilly	119 (124)	93

Source: Citeline (2015)

Appendix 2: List of Big Data Congresses

Big Data Events for Pharma (Search strings: "big data pharma industry", "big data congress pharma")

Congress	Results found
Pharma Data Analytics http://www.bigdatainpharma.com/ 29 September – 1 October 2014 (Brussels, Belgium)	✓
Big Data in Pharma http://www.smi-online.co.uk/pharmaceuticals/uk/conference/Big-Data-in-Pharma 12-13 May 2014 (London, UK)	✓
Big Data & Analytics for Pharma Summit https://theinnovationenterprise.com/summits/big-data-analytics-for-pharma-summit-philadelphia-November-2015 4-5 November 2015 (Philadelphia, USA)	✓
Big Data & Analytics in Healthcare Summit http://www.theinnovationenterprise.com/summits/bigdata-healthcare-philadelphia-2015 13-14 May 2015 (Philadelphia, USA)	x
Big DIP Europe http://bigdatapharma-europe.com/ 27-29 January 2015 (London, UK)	✓
Big DIP USA http://big-datapharma.com/ 22-24 September 2015 (Boston, USA)	✓
Oxford Global Annual Pharmaceutical IT Congress http://www.pharmatechnology-summit.com 23-24 September 2015 (London, UK)	✓
Oxford Global Pharmaceutical IT World Asia Congress http://www.pharmaitasia-congress.com 25-26 March 2014 (Singapore)	✓
Medizin Innovativ – Med Tech Pharma http://www.medtech-pharma.de/deutsch/veranstaltungen/kongress/kongress-2014/programm/big-data-management---analytics.aspx 2 -3 July 2014 (Nuremberg, Germany)	x
Pharmaceutical Management Science Association Annual Conference http://www.pmsa.net/conferences/2015-annual-conference 19-22 April 2015 (Airlington, USA)	x

Big Data in Clinical Development 2015 http://www.bigdataleadersforum.com 7-8 October 2015 (Washington DC, 2015)	✓
Cambridge Healthtech Institute's Seventh Annual Integrated Pharma Informatics & Data Science http://www.triconference.com/Integrated-Pharma-Informatics/ 16-18 February 2015 (San Francisco, USA)	✓
Fleming Europe Pharma Exabyte http://pharma.flemingeurope.com/pharma-exabyte-conference/program 27-28 May 2015 (Berlin, Germany)	✓
Marcus Evans Annual Pharma Data Analytics http://www.marcusevans-conferences-northamerican.com/marcusevans-conferences-event-details.asp?EventID=21511#.VSKiyboWlW8 18-19 November 2014 (Philadelphia, USA)	✓
Bio Data World Congress http://www.healthnetworkcommunications.com/conference/biodata/ 21-22 October 2015 (Cambridge, USA)	✓
Big Data in Healthcare http://bigdata-healthcare.com 28-30 April 2015 (Boston, USA)	x
informs Healthcare 2015 http://meetings2.informs.org/wordpress/healthcare2015/ 29-31 July 2015 (Nashville, USA)	x
Big Data in Pharma 2015 http://recunnect.com/pharma-events/big-data-in-pharma-2015/ 17 June 2015 (London, UK)	✓
Digital Communication in Healthcare http://www.euroforum.de/veranstaltungen/digital_communication_in_healthcare_juli2015 7/8 July 2015 (Frankfurt/Main, Germany)	x
World BioPharma Big Data Congress http://www.terrapinn.com/conference/biopharmabigdata/index.stm 4-5 March 2014 (London, UK)	x
Bio IT World Conference & EXPO'15 http://www.bio-itworldexpo.com/Drug-Discovery-Informatics/ 21-23 April 2015 (Boston, USA)	✓
The Pharmaceutical Strategy Conference http://www.iirusa.com/pharmastrategic/home.xml 29 September – 1 October 2014 (New York, USA)	✓
Big Data in Biomedicine https://bigdata.stanford.edu 20-22 May 2015 (Stanford, USA)	x

Cambridge's Healthtech Institute's Biomarker & Diagnostics World Congress http://www.biomarkerworldcongress.com/Big-Data-Biomarkers/ 5-7 May 2015 (Philadelphia, USA)	✓
Personalised Cancer Medicine & Big Data Analysis http://www.nature.com/natureevents/science/events/30817Personalised_Cancer_Medicine_Big_Data_Analysis_7th_International_Conference_of_Contemporary_Oncology 25-27 March 2015 (Poznan, Poland)	x
BioPharma Asia Convention 2015 http://www.terrapinn.com/exhibition/bio-asia/index.stm?_ga=1.104219328.158402373.1428337859 23-25 March 2015 (Singapore)	x
Advances in NGS & Big Data http://selectbiosciences.com/conferences/index.aspx?conf=NGSBD2014 14-15 May 2014 (Barcelona, Spain)	x
Real World Evidence & Data Partnerships Summit http://www.eyeforpharma.com/real-world-data-and-health-outcomes/conference-agenda.php 14-15 October 2014 (Bethesda, USA)	✓
Predictive Analytics World for Healthcare http://www.predictiveanalyticsworld.com/health/2015/ 27 September – 1 October, 2015 (Boston, USA)	✓

Health Innovation Congresses (Search string: "healthcare innovation conference", ""healthcare innovation congress")

Congress	Results found
The Pharmaceutical Strategy Conference http://www.iirusa.com/pharmastrategic/home.xml 29 September – 1 October 2014 (New York, USA)	x
Global Health & Innovation Conference http://www.uniteforsight.org/conference/ 28-29 March 2015 (New Haven, USA)	x
Forbes Healthcare Summit http://www.forbes.com/healthcare-summit/ 2-3 December 2015 (New York City, USA)	x

General Big Data Events (Search string: "big data summit")

Congress	Results found
Big Data Innovation Summit https://theinnovationenterprise.com/summits/big-data-innovation-summit-san-jose/speakers 28-29 April 2015 (San José, USA)	x
BITKOM Big Data Summit http://www.bitkom-bigdata.de 25 February 2015 (Hanau, Germany)	x
Big Data Innovation https://theinnovationenterprise.com/summits/big-data-innovation-boston-2015 23-24 September 2015 (Boston, USA)	x
Big Data & Analytics Innovation Summit https://theinnovationenterprise.com/summits/big-data-analytics-innovation-summit-london-2015 15-16 October 2015 (London, UK)	x
Big Data Summit http://www.bigdatasummit.us 17-19 May 2015 (Atlanta, USA)	x
Big Data & Analytics Summit 2015 http://www.computingsummit.com/bigdata/static/speakers 26 March 2015 (London, UK)	x
Smart Data Summit 2015 http://www.bigdata-me.com 25-26 May 2015 (Dubai, UAE)	x
Leverage Big Data '15 http://www.leveragebigdata.com 16-18 March 2015 (Ponte Vedra Beach, USA)	x
Data Summit http://www.dbta.com/DataSummit/2015/ 11-13 May 2015 (New York, USA)	x
SMART DATA Summit http://www.smart-data-summit.de 7-8 December 2015 (Hamburg, Germany)	x
Cloud & Big Data Summit http://www.con-nect.com.au/cloudandbigdata.html 22 April 2015 (Melbourne, Australia)	x
TELCO Big Data Summit http://usa.telcobigdata.com 9 September 2015 (Las Vegas, USA)	x

Supernova – the Big Data Summit http://www.quantcastsupernova-eu.com 23 October 2014 (London, UK)	x
RSM Leadership Summit 2014 http://www.rsm.nl/rsm-leadership-summit-2014/ 3 October 2014 (Rotterdam, The Netherlands)	x
IP EXPO Europe http://www.ipexpo.co.uk/Big-Data-Evolution-Summit 8-9 October 2014 (London, UK)	x
Nasscom Big Data and Analytics Summit http://www.nasscom.in/bigdata 27 June 2014 (Hyderabad, India)	x
IEEE Big Data Congress http://www.ieeebigdata.org/2015/ 27 June – 2 July 2015 (New York, USA)	x
Cloud World Forum http://analyticsandbigdatacongress.com 24-25 June 2015 (London, UK)	x

Appendix 3: Detailed results - online research on presence at congresses

Novartis:

Name of congress	Insights
Big Data Events for Pharma (Google search strings: "big data congress pharma"; "big data conference pharma"; "big data summit pharma")	

Big Data in Pharma 12-13 May 2014 (London, UK)	• **Presentation: Leveraging Big Data To Study Comparative Effectiveness Research (CER): A Case Example in Multiple Sclerosis** *(Niklas Bergvall, Senior Director, Global HEOR Neuroscience, Novartis Pharmaceuticals)*
	  o Developing a systematic approach for identifying CER opportunities for pharma
	  o MS is a complex, chronic disease that requires monitoring of real-world effectiveness to inform clinical and economic decision-making.
	  o The use of data from multiple sources can overcome the limitations associated with assessing outcomes using a single source of information, such as individual database or registry studies.
	  o This combination of data sources provides useful critical information on real-world outcomes in a general MS population that can be used to complement data from clinical trials and observational studies in MS
	• **Presentation: Leveraging Existing Data From Legacy Clinical Trials** *(Pantaleo Nacci, Head Statistical Reporting, Novartis Limited)*
	  o Discover a goldmine at your fingertips
	  o Understanding how to prepare it for use
	  o Choice of a (set of) standard(s)
	  o Evaluating future developments
	• **Shared Presentation: Lessons Learned So Far! Understanding Big Data And Its Uses For The Pharmaceutical World** *(Pantaleo Nacci, Head Statistical Reporting, Novartis Limited)*
	  o What has been learned
	  o Evaluating what has and hasn't worked
	  o What are the next steps in the big data strategy

Oxford Global Annual Pharmaceutical IT Congress 23-24 September 2015 (London, UK)	• Speakers:
	  o Dimitrios Georgiopoulos, Chief Scientific Officer UK
	  o Philippe Marc, Global Head of Preclinical Informatics, Novartis Institutes for Biomedical Research

Oxford Global Pharmaceutical IT World Asia Congress
25-26 March 2014
(Singapore)
	• Speakers:
	   o Stephen Elms, Head of Automation & IT, Biopharmaceutical Operations Singapore, Novartis
	   o Dinesh Pillaipakkamnatt, Global Head, Central Analytics Function

Fleming Europe Pharma Exabyte 27-28 May 2015 (Berlin, Germany)	• Speakers: Edward Oakeley, Basel Head, Next Generation Sequencing Technologies

Bio Data World Congress
21-22 October 2015
(Cambridge, USA)
	• **Presentation: The current and future status of ultra-long read sequencing studies** *(Edward Oakeley, Basel Head, Next Generation Sequencing Technologies)*
	   o The challenge of providing information over length scales large enough to reveal genome structural variants
	   o Benefits and limitations of the key ultra-long read sequencing platforms
	   o With improvements in throughput, what do the platforms need to offer to keep pace with the developments?

Big Data in Pharma 2015
17 June 2015
(London, UK)
	• **Presentation: Big Data in Clinical Trials: An Experience in Vaccines** *(Pantaleo Nacci, Head of Statistical Safety & Epidemiology/PV, Novartis)*
	   o Benefits of data standardization
	   o Data visualisation and safety signalling
	   o Regulatory submission support

Bio IT World Conference & EXPO 21-23 April 2015 (Boston, USA)	• **Workshop: Predictive Analytics** - Instructors among other representatives (Exaptve, GNS Healthcare, Tamr): *Mark Burfoot – Global Head, Knowledge Office, Novartis Institutes for BioMedical Research* Dr. Burfoot is the Global Head of the Knowledge Office, which reports into the Program Office for NIBR. This includes the NIBR Competitive Intelligence Group and the Novartis Knowledge Center, which provides key global resources and services to Novartis. Dr. Burfoot joined NIBR in early 2009 moving from being the global lead for Information Services at Pfizer for research, development and commercial activities.

Pfizer:

Name of congress	Insights
Big Data Events for Pharma (Google search strings: "big data congress pharma"; "big data conference pharma"; "big data summit pharma")	
Pharma Data Analytics 29 September – 1 October 2014 (Brussels, Belgium)	• Gerhard Noelken, Business IT Lead, member of congress advisory board
Big Data & Analytics for Pharma Summit 4-5 November 2015 (Philadelphia, USA)	• **Speaker: Catherine Marshall, Director, Information Strategy & Analytics (Presentation to be confirmed)** Cathy is an Information Strategist in the Clinical Informatics & Innovations Group at Pfizer. She has been with Pfizer for 9 years and has focused extensively on data integration, discoverability, and search in order to enable decision support in the Drug Discovery and Development Process. For the last two years, she has been working on a project at Pfizer to establish a clinical data strategy to enable precision medicine research from very early drug discovery through patient selection in the clinical trials process.
Big DIP Europe 27-29 January 2015 (London, UK)	• **Chairman at the Congress: Josephine A. Sallono, Vice President, Outcomes & Evidence, Global Health and Value** Josephine Sollano is the Vice President of the Outcomes & Evidence (O&E) Team within the Global Health and Value Organization for Pfizer, Inc. In her current role, Jo leads a large team responsible for value evidence generation across the Pfizer portfolio to facilitate pricing, reimbursement, and patient access to medicines. Using highly advanced methodologies and study designs, the O&E team utilizes real world and clinical trial data to generate evidence specific to payor, regulatory, prescriber, patient, and policymaker's needs.
Big DIP USA 22-24 September 2014 (Boston, USA)	• Sample speaker: Marc Berger, Vice President, Real World Data & Analytics
Oxford Global Annual Pharmaceutical IT Congress 23-24 September 2015 (London, UK)	• Speaker: 　o Marc Berger, Vice President, Real World Data & Analytics 　o Gerhard Noelken, Global Business IT Lead for Pharmaceutical Science, Pfizer WRD 　o Sergio H. Rotstein, Director, Research Business Technology 　o Q&A: Marc Berger, Vice President, Real World Data & Ana-

	lytics

Oxford Global Pharmaceutical IT World Asia Congress
25-26 March 2014
(Singapore)
	• Speaker:
	   ◦ Jay Bergeron, Director, Translational and Bioinformatics
	   ◦ Gerhard Noelken, Global Business IT Lead for Pharmaceutical Science

Cambridge Healthtech Institute's Seventh Annual Integrated Pharma Informatics & Data Science 16- 18 February 2015 (San Francisco, USA)	• **Presentation: Using Informatics to Enable Precision Medicine in Oncology** *(Susie Stephens, Senior Director, Oncology & West Coast IT, Pfizer)* ◦ Successfully enabling precision medicine for oncology requires a robust strategy for working with data, implementing analysis pipelines, and sharing results of analyses with scientists. This presentation highlights capabilities that have been enabled in these areas through a close collaboration between Oncology Research and Research IT.
Fleming Europe Pharma Exabyte 27-28 May 2015 (Berlin, Germany)	• Speakers: Jerry Lanfear, Head of Research Business Technologies
Marcus Evans Annual Pharma Data Analytics 18-19 November 2014 (Philadelphia, USA)	• Speaker: Aaron Galaznik, MD, MBA, Senior Director, Real World Data and Analytics, Global Health and Value

Bio Data World Congress
21-22 October 2015
(Cambridge, USA)
	• **Presentation: NGS and the discovery of causative genes for pain** *(Dr. Ciara Vangjeli, Associate Director and Senior Applied Geneticist)*
	   ◦ Therapeutic opportunities identified through genetic studies of rare pain disorders
	   ◦ The use of NGS to identify causative genes for pain
	   ◦ Results, challenges and further work

Bio IT World Conference & EXPO 21-23 April 2015 (Boston, USA)	*Clinical & Translational Informatics* • **Presentation: Technology Framework to Operationalize Biomarker-Focused Clinical Research** *(Brenda Yanak, Ph.D., Director, Precision Medicine Leader, Clinical Innovation, Pfizer)* *Data Visualization and Exploration Tools* • **Presentation: Toward an Open Source Suite to Bridge the Gap between Plate-Based Screening and Results** *(Peter Henstock, Ph.D., Senior Principal Scientist, Research Business Technology Group, Pfizer, Inc.)*

o Scientists in academic laboratories through large pharmaceutical companies have all encountered the challenges of efficiently extracting results from plate-based assay data. Issues from compound/reagent/plate management, assay format variability, instrumentation, output file formats, and analysis software invariably lead to a cumbersome process. To improve the efficiency, an open source suite of web-based tools is being developed that spans the key steps of plate editing, QC/QA calculation and visualization, and a user-driven non-coding approach to output file parsing. For results analysis, the suite includes visualization and computational approaches for interactively interpreting single-point, dose-response, and multivariate data.

Collaborations and Open Access Innovations
- **Presentation: Imitation and Disruption: Impact on Open Source Software Success in the Life Sciences** (*Jay Bergeron, Director, Translational and Bioinformatics, Pfizer, Inc.*)
- There are many successful examples of open source software (OSS) both within and outside of the life sciences community. However, investigators sponsoring software-based efforts need to consider many factors, including resourcing, architecture fragmentation, maintenance and their customer community when selecting between commercial and open license alternatives. This presentation will review such factors. Motivations that give rise to voluntary participation, by software developers, in OSS projects have been well analyzed. Socio-Psychological factors that include the potential for individual development and personal recognition, as well as the opportunity to contribute to self-selected high value efforts, have been promoted as drivers of OSS contribution. Substantial work has been conducted to relate architectural elements with the free-rider tolerance that is associated with successful OSS initiatives. However, empirical evidence to support the hypothesized relationship between architecture and OSS participation is limited. Moreover, the extent to which Socio-Psychological factors promote OSS participation is difficult to quantify given substantial OSS investments that are provided by government and commercial enterprises. Additionally, open source licensing models may not preclude commercial extension, packaging and consultancies. To extend the traditional dialog regarding OSS implementation, imitation of existing business patterns and discretionary pricing models that enable under-served customers, leading to market disruption, are considered as key drivers of OSS success.

	- Panel discussion: Finding Innovation in Collaboration Environments: Documentum SharePoint, Veeva, and Tigers, Oh My! (*Instructor among other representatives from Biogen, AstraZeneca, J&J: Jay Bergeron, Direcor, Translational & Bioninformatics, Pfizer, Inc.*)
	  o Topics to be covered include:
	    ▪ Driving Internal Collaborations
	    ▪ Enabling Global Project Teams
	    ▪ Enabling Precompetitive Collaboration
	    ▪ Addressing the Challenge of Externalization
	    ▪ Enabling Collaboration with Partners
	    ▪ Collaborative Business Models
	  o Jay's team is responsible for informatics support for Clinical Research and Precision Medicine. He is also the Scientific Coordinator of eTRIKS (European Translational Research and Information Knowledge Management Services), a 23M Euro program to support translational data management for the IMI that uses Open Source Software (tranSMART) as the core system. Also, he co-leads the code committee of the tranSMART Foundation, a non-profit community organizer for the Open Source tranSMART application

Cambridge's Healthtech Institute's Biomarker & Diagnostics World Congress 5-7 May 2015 (Philadelphia, USA)	- Presentation: Using Clinical and Real World Data for Biomarker Discovery in Precision Medicine (*Joan Sopczynski, Ph.D., Senior Manager, Predictive Informatics, Business Insights, R&D Business Technology, Pfizer*) o Real world and clinical trial databases consist of large patient data sets that can be explored for biological insights. Examples will be presented describing the analysis of this patient data for biomarker identification and disease knowledge. Methods used to analyze the data, including the application of machine learning techniques, will be described highlighting their ability to identify biomarkers distinguishing patient populations.

Real World Evidence & Data Partnerships Summit
14-15 October 2014
(Bethesda, USA)
	- Pharma Case Study: Leveraging Real World Data to Inform Decision-Making on a Timely Basis (*Marc Berger, Vice President, Real World Data & Analytics*)
	  o Realize that Big Data vs. Little data is less important than whether you are systematically gaining insights from the data you have
	  o Hear why most organizations do not derive the full value from the data assets they have access to
	  o As asking sharp questions is hard, learn about rapid cycle analysis that decision makers need interactive support through
	  o Understand that RW Data is improving but may not be rich

		enough currently to benefit from machine learning/advanced analytics
Predictive Analytics World for Healthcare 27 September – 1 October 2015 (Boston, USA)	•	**Case Study: Crowdsourcing Predictive Analytics to Enhance Clinical Trial Design** *(Scott Jelinski, Principal Research Scientist)* ○ As part of Pfizer's open innovation initiative, we have been experimenting with different techniques to develop algorithms to solve tough analytic questions. Here we access the collective knowledge of the "crowd" to develop innovative and novel solutions to analytical questions associated with "big data" including patient level medical data. We will share a case study where we have crowdsourced predictive models to identify patients who are likely to have progressive disease symptoms. We will share the pros and cons of our approach and outline situations in which crowdsourcing may be an alternative approach to other more traditional activities.

Sanofi:

Name of congress	Insights
Big Data Events for Pharma (Google search strings: "big data congress pharma"; "big data conference pharma"; "big data summit pharma")	
Big DIP Europe 27-29 January 2015 (London, UK)	• **Presentation: Innovative Partnering for Holistic Results: Who, Why & How** *(Charles Gerrits, Vice President, Early Patient & Medical Perspectives, Sanofi)* • **Presentation: Taking the Plunge into Web-Based Pharmacovigilance and Signal Detection** *(Marie-Laure Kurzinger, Epidemiologist – Associate Director, Sanofi)* • **Panel discussion: What's Holding us Back When it Comes to Social Media Listening?** *(Panelist: Marie-Laure Kurzinger, Epidemiologist – Associate Director, Sanofi)* • **Publication: Real World Product Design using Real World Data** (Usman Iqbal, Senior Director, Head of Oncology, Evidence & Value Development)

Oxford Global Annual Pharmaceutical IT Congress 23-24 September 2015 (London, UK)	• Speakers:
	  o James Connelly, Global Head, Research Data Management
	  o Brian Ellerman (Head of Technology Scouting and Information Science Innovation, Sanofi)
	  o Charles Gerrits, Innovative Patient-Centric Endpoints and Solutions

Big Data in Clinical Development 2015 7-8 October 2015 (Washington DC, USA)	• **Presentation: How the cloud is overcoming the problems of distance and data size in clinical trials** *(Rhett Alden, Senior Director, Cloud)*
	  o Overcoming challenges of security, access management and cost efficiencies
	  o Establishing large-scale flexible infrastructures
	• **Presentation: The value of Big Data: how analytics differentiates winners** *(Dr. William Daley, VP, Medical Affairs, Aging, Business Development & Licensing)*
	  o Tracking the emergence of pragmatic clinical trials to leverage big data resources
	  o Can you turn an observational trial into a clinical trial?
	  o Pragmatic trials – to be run in parallel with clinical trials?
	  o Adaptive trials – how can big data support and strengthen their value?
	• **Presentation: Finding the data: patients as partners in medi-**

	cines development (Francis Rienzo, Vice President of Partners in Patient Health)
	    o The patient's role and experience in big data collection and utilization
	    o What patient advocates and patients can do to advance the practice of personalized medicine

Roche:

Name of congress	Insights
Big Data Events for Pharma (Google search strings: "big data congress pharma"; "big data conference pharma"; "big data summit pharma")	
Oxford Global Annual Pharmaceutical IT Congress 23-24 September 2015 (London, UK)	• Speakers: ○ Michael Braxenthaler, Pharma Research and Early Development Informatics, Global Head Strategic Alliances ○ Juergen Hammer (Global Head Data Science, Center Head Pharma Research and Early Development Informatics)
Oxford Global Pharmaceutical IT World Asia Congress 25-26 March 2014 (Singapore)	• Speakers: ○ Michael Braxenthaler, Pharma Research and Early Development Informatics, Global Head Strategic Alliances ○ Juergen Hammer, Global Head Disease and Translational Informatics ○ Alain Nanzer, Global Area Head Non-Clinical Safety Informatics ○ Paul Whitehead, pRED Informatics Center Head
Big Data in Clinical Development 2015 7-8 October 2015 (Washington DC, USA)	• **Presentation: Image-based biomarkers to enhance clinical research** *(Dr. Angelika Fuchs, Senor Data Scientist, pRED Informatics)* ○ Challenges and opportunities of integrating tissue-based imaging data with genomic data ○ Bringing tissue-centric biomarker data to clinical teams for decision making
Cambridge Healthtech Institute's Seventh Annual Integrated Pharma Informatics & Data Science 16- 18 February 2015 (San Francisco, USA)	• **Presentation: Experience & Challenges of Creating and Implementing a Data Science Function** *(Juergen Hammer, Ph.D., MBA, Roche Pharmaceutical Research and Early Development; Center Head, Informatics/IT; Global Head, Data Science, Roche Innovation Center New York)* The Data Scientist profession has been named "The Sexiest Job of the 21st Century" and is often considered an essential component of Big Data Analytics. However, the Data Scientist Function in Pharma and Biotech is far from being established. I will discuss the organizational positioning of our multi-capability Data Science teams, how we measure performance, and which cultural shifts are required to maximize the impact of Data Science on the drug pipeline. I will provide a number of Data Science examples highlighting the importance of this function in bridging the gap between massive content and end-user decision making in a world of deficient

	Application Landscapes

Bio IT World Conference & EXPO
21-23 April 2015
(Boston, USA)
	Workshop: Biologics, Bioassay, and Biospecimen Registration Systems:
	• **Presentation: Semantic Backbone for Integrating Biological Registration Systems** (*Martin Romacker, Senior Scientist, Data and Information Architecture, Roche Innovation Center Basel*)
	    o Data Science heavily builds on semantic integration and flexible data federation. The integration of highly diverse external repositories constitutes the major challenge. In pRED (Pharma Research and Early Development) at Roche, we take a very principled approach to data management building on a centralized knowledge hub. The knowledge hub provides controlled terminologies for biological registration systems (such as for cell lines) and underpins the data curation process for scientific content leading to correct, complete and coherent data. As a result, we create a shared reference layer for internal and external data forming a growing knowledge graph based on standards driven by Pistoia, IMI or W3C.
	• **Presentation: Molecular Registration of Novel and Complex Biologics** (*Rudolf Kinder, Senior Scientist, Roche Innovation Center Penzberg*)
	    o The increasing complexity of novel biological drugs enforces the development of supporting software systems. This presentation will showcase how the last year's awarded HELM Notation fuels a full-blown registration system. The new TaPIR platform at Roche enables the registration of all kind of complex molecules including conjugates with small molecules, Toxins or RNA. Automated detection of protein features like mutations, formats (CrossMab, scFAB) ensure a high registration quality and a smooth user experience.
	• **Presentation: Automated Registration and Visualization of Complex Therapeutic Proteins** (*Clemens Wrzodek, Ph.D., Scientific Software Engineer, Technical Project Manager, Roche Diagnostics GmbH*)
	    o Registration of complex proteins, e.g., antibodies, at molecular level is a sophisticated process. We have extended our established registration procedures to be ready for high-throughput sequencing data. Therefore, template-based bulk operations have been developed for Roche researches that allow them to register hundreds of antibodies with a single click. In order to allow the users a quick verification of what has been registered, the system automatically gener-

ates visualizations of the proteins by depicting the chains with their domains and drawing the connections between them (using an enhanced version of the Pistoia HELM editor).
- **Presentation: Rapid Integration of Cancer Genomics Data Using Hadoop and Cloudera's Impala** (*Sittichoke Saisanit, Ph.D., Data Scientist, Informatics, Pharmaceutical Research and Early Development Informatics, Roche Innovation Center New York*)
    - We explored Cloudera Impala for analysis of cancer genomics data. Without data transformation and reformatting, Impala tables can be created quickly from files on Hadoop file system with a simple command. Such speed and flexibility enable us to interrogate data without spending much time on schema design, index creation, query tuning and data cleaning. Impala can be accessed through Spotfire allowing flexibility of data visualization.

Bioinformatics
- **Presentation: Streamlined Planning, Execution, Data Capture and Analysis of Peptide Pre-formulation Stability Studies** (*Roman Affentranger, Dr. sc. Nat, Head, Small Molecule Discovery Workflows, Roche*)
    - The presentation will illustrate what we have implemented for the peptide pre-formulation scientists in their electronic lab notebook to efficiently design peptide formulation stability studies. The study can cover a number of different formulations, and with the definition of time points, stress conditions and desired analytical methods the required number of vials as well as individual material amounts are automatically calculated. Individual analytical results are captured through predesigned templates that are specific for the different types or analytics, and the results are linked to the stability study by a unique study ID. All along the study execution, as well as for the completed study, all the data -- formulation composition, study design and all analytical results - are pulled together in a data analysis tool, also within the electronic lab notebook. The data analysis tool allows selection of individual or multiple formulations, time points, and stress points, and therefore offers unique insights which greatly support decision making for improved formulation design.

Software Development
- **Presentation: Semantic Integration of Unstructured Safety Study Data: Experiences and Outlook** (*Alain Nanzer, Ph.D., Global Head Safety & Development Workflows, Pharma Research and Early Development Informatics, Roche Innovation Center Basel*)
  - In pharmaceutical R&D vast amounts of study data are generated -- in house and externally -- which are used to advance drug projects and then end as reports in document management systems or on file shares. Most often these data are lost for further scientific analysis, as no structured search and access is possible. Common approaches to load such data to scientific data warehouses require complex ETL processes to normalize the results, are very labor intensive and not well suited for large sets of unstructured legacy data. The presentation will share our experiences implementing a platform using semantic integration technologies to provide scientists search, evaluation, and advanced visualization capabilities for safety in vivo study data. Furthermore we will show how the platform has been extended providing fast access to real-time study data, and then evolved to a data turntable for external study data and submissions to regulatory authorities.

Next-Generation Sequencing Informatics
- **Presentation: Deep Sequencing Based Analysis of Ig repertoire in Humanized Mice** (*Stefan Klostermann, Ph.D., Expert Scientist, Bioinformatics/Data Science, Roche Innovation Center Penzeberg*)
  - On our quest for human biotherapeutical antibodies we developed a novel methodology: Instead of replacing the mouse genomic immune loci by the human orthologs we reconstituted the humoral immune response in immunodeficient mice transplanted with human hematopoietic stem cells. An in-depth characterization of the reconstituted immune system by data analysis of deep sequencing Ig repertoire validated the humanized mouse be immunological equivalent to human donors.

Data Visualization and Exploration Tools
- **Presentation: Bringing Process, Chemical & Analytical Data Together: Data Mining & Visualization** (*Jean-Michel Adam, Ph.D., Senior Principal Scientist, Preclinical CMC Process Research, Roche Pharma Research & Early Development, Roche Innovation Center Basel*)

- Automated reactors, coupled with in-/off-line analytical tools, are routinely used in the chemical process R&D world. While these do help increase process knowledge and overall productivity, an increasing amount of data are being generated, generally in a fragmented way. We would like to report a first approach aiming at integrating process data from automated reactors, analytical systems output as well as chemical information from Electronic Lab Notebook.

Workshop: The Impact of research informatics on laboratory evolution

- The advancements in technology have significantly changed how we work today. This workshop will introduce you to the fundamentals of some technologies and where we see it evolving. It is meant to be highly interactive and we encourage you to provide you point of view, participation and feedback.

Have you ever wondered how the increasing changes in technology will change our working environments? We will address technologies for laboratory and office use. This will focus on those technologies which are productive and those with a high potential to be disruptive to your organizations. Topics covered will include a look at how early technologies like wearables, full 3D immersive, 3D printing, Gestures, Surface and Digital Holography will change how we interact with our computers, systems and applications. The concept of "data at your fingertips" is no longer a vision but a reality today.

We will target how these technologies affect traditional IT organizations and the need to adapt in order to allow advancements and provide agility. The agility is required in the labs and office environments and the line between these environments has become clouded. Key topics to challenge will be computing, storage and networks as well as collaboration tools and additional infrastructure needs. This will mean as IT organizations we will need to narrow the ever growing gaps between traditional Corporate IT and Research IT and identify where synergies exits and partnerships are necessary. Discussions on how to change and influence these areas within your organizations is a must and should be happening today.

- Instructors:

  Javier A. Roa, Global Head of Technical Operations & Research Infrastructure:

  Javier A. Roa, is the Global Head of Technical Operations & Research infrastructure for F. Hoffmann-La Roche, Ltd. located in Basel Switzerland. Roche is a pioneer in healthcare for nearly 120 years. He is a technologist by training and computer engineer interested in applying innovative technologies in Research. He has 27 years' experience in the Pharmaceutical industry and currently leads global teams in N.Y., Shanghai, Switzerland and Germany. He is also responsible for the High Performance Computing transformation initiative at Roche and leads the Informatics Communication Technologies - ICT initiative at the Global Roche Innovation Centers.

Mischa J. Huber, Basel Head of Technical Operations & Research Infrastructure:

Mischa J. Huber, is the Basel Head of Technical Operations & Research Infrastructure for F. Hoffmann-La Roche, Ltd. located in Basel Switzerland. He started his career as a laboratory technician by training and has been looking over and caring for these environments ever since. He transitioned his career into IT where he saw the need to bring key innovations to scientist hands and the needs for automation and data accessibility. He currently focuses much of his work on how to improve work in research laboratory with innovative solutions. He has 22 years' experience in the Pharmaceutical industry and currently leads a local team in Basel. In addition he is also a Technical Project Manager within the Research informatics organization.

Alexander Rossi, Basel Head Laboratory Information Systems & Support:

Alexander Rossi is leading the global laboratory information systems & support teams for F.Hoffmann- La-Roche, Ltd. Basel Switzerland. He has over 15 years of experience in Pharmaceutical Industry with focus on IT Infrastructure and Laboratory technologies. Leader of several Global projects, Team Leads and Service Management within Biomedical Research & Development and Global IT infrastructure. Delivery of international environments possessing successful track record of team building, system migration, hightech projects (infrastructure, software, network, data centers) and quality improvement projects.

Cambridge's Healthtech Institute's Biomarker & Diagnostics World Congress 5-7 May 2015 (Philadelphia, USA)	• **Presentation: Applying Data Science in Translational Clinical Research** *(James Cai, Ph.D., Head, Data Science, Roche)* The intelligent use of Big Data has transformed many industries. It also presents numerous opportunities for pharmaceutical companies as we collect more genomic Big Data directly from patients. In this talk I will outline a Data Science model that emphasizes mixed-capability teams and impact on science and business decisions. I will discuss how quantitative analytical skills, agile programming, novel technologies and business acumen all contribute to this model. I will illustrate with examples where Data Science was applied to clinical research resulting in new scientific insights and better business decisions.

Merck & Co:

Name of congress	Insights
Big Data Events for Pharma (Google search strings: "big data congress pharma"; "big data conference pharma"; "big data summit pharma")	

Pharma Data Analytics
29 September – 1 October 2014
(Brussels, Belgium)
	• Presentation: Exploring Different Methods of Data Mapping: The platform integration challenge for "Going Paperless": an experience report from the veterinarian GxP area *(Brunhilde Schoelzke, Senior Specialist, R&D Analytics & Data)*
	    o Effective ways of mapping data to aid in analyzing data
	    o Enabling access to information in standard formats
	    o Identifying best practices in data mapping

Big Data & Analytics for Pharma Summit 4-5 November 2015 (Philadelphia, USA)	• **Speaker: Barnaby Fountain, Director, Business Analytics Realization (Presentation to be confirmed)** A certified Master Black Belt and Change Agent, Barney has over 14 years of experience executing transformational continuous improvement strategies in large organizations. He's currently responsible for driving benefits realization of the IT analytics portfolio to meet/exceed their $1.3B target. In this role, he ensures analytics projects deliver value, architects cross-functional strategic projects, and advances the use of data analytics to run the business more effectively. Prior to joining Merck in 2007, Barney managed process improvement strategies in Honeywell's Global Business Services organization as a Black Belt and IT Program Manager. • **Speaker: Laura Galuchie, Director, Clinical Performance, Analytics & Innovation (Presentation to be confirmed)** Laura leads a newly reconfigured team focused on providing clinical trial operational data back to the organization. Internal customers range from trial team members who manage ongoing trials to senior management who digest the various analyses to understand the impact of process improvement initiatives and identify areas for focus. Laura spent most of her career as a consumer of information– from CRA to Therapeutic Area Clinical Operational Lead - and is able to use that experience in guiding new data analyses and interactive tool development. • **Speaker: Julia O'Neill, Director, Engineering (Presentation to be confirmed)** Julia O'Neill, Director in Global Science, Technology & Commercialization, is responsible for process robustness strategy and monitoring for Merck manufacturing. Her team integrates data management and analytic expertise with process knowledge, to identify

Big DIP USA 22-24 September 2014 (Boston, USA)	• Sample Speaker: Sachin Jain, Chief Medical Information & Innovation Officer

Oxford Global Annual Pharmaceutical IT Congress
23-24 September 2015
(London, UK)
	• Speakers:
	   o Jan Hauss, Head Central Analytics Informatics
	   o Dermot McCaul, Director, Preclinical Development and Biologics IT
	   o Andrew Porter, Director, Enterprise Architecture
	   o Martin Ryzl, Director, GIC Analytics Platform Engineering

Oxford Global Pharmaceutical IT World Asia Congress 25-26 March 2014 (Singapore)	• Speakers: o Eike Staub, Computational Biologist, Merck

Big Data in Clinical Development 2015
7-8 October 2015
(Washington DC, USA)
	• **Presentation: Generating real world evidence and leveraging it to inform clinical trial design, render better decisions and reduce the cost of care** *(Dr. Thomas Tsang, Chief Medical Officer, Merck Healthcare Services and Solution)*
	   o Structured and unstructured data sources – how are trusted 3rd parties capturing and aggregating the data, and guaranteeing quality
	   o Developing national registries and linking to claims data to track outcomes
	   o How soon will genetics/genomics be combined with EHRs at a larger scale?
	   o How do you prove the ROI? How do...
	• **Keynote – Lecture: Real world data science innovation - where in the product lifecycle will big data have greatest impact, utility and value?** *(Roy D. Baynes, MD, PhD, Senior Vice President Global Clinical Development, Merck Research Laboratories)*
	   o Impact on discovery, development, commercial, post-marketing
	   o Are we asking the right questions of all the data?
	   o Is the use of big data to prove or disprove a hypothesis ready for prime time?
	   o Building a hierarchy of real world evidence – how will big data help us get there?
	• **Panel discussion between heads of clinical development from pharma, biotech and cros** *(Panelist: Roy D. Baynes, MD, PhD, Sen-*

	ior Vice President Global Clinical Development) ○ What infrastructure is required to allow the capture, integration and end-to-end flow of data throughout the pharma organization? ○ Driving internal collaboration and interpretation skills so that everyone speaks a common language – including at leadership level ○ Who is best positioned to interrogate the plethora of data and ask the right...
Cambridge Healthtech Institute's Seventh Annual Integrated Pharma Informatics & Data Science 16- 18 February 2015 (San Francisco, USA)	• **Presentation: Enabling Secure Real World Data Exchange and Collaborative Analytics across Healthcare Organizations** *(Patrick Loerch, Director, Health IT, Information Technology)* ○ Healthcare reform, the decline in the price of genome sequencing and growing pressures from government and payers to demonstrate the effectiveness of novel therapies are creating a new market centered on access to real world data. The increasing economic pressures of this rapidly growing market are colliding with the need to ensure the security of patient data. We have developed, proven out and executed on a novel approach to enabling the secure sharing and collaborative analysis of real world data across healthcare organizations. As a representative of one of the core consumer bases of the secondary use of real world data we are introducing new modality for secure information exchange and collaborative analytics that benefits and meets the security needs of diverse healthcare organizations.
Fleming Europe Pharma Exabyte 27-28 May 2015 (Berlin, Germany)	• Speaker: Martin Ryzl, Director, GIC Analytics Platform Engineering
Marcus Evans Annual Pharma Data Analytics 18-19 November 2014 (Philadelphia, USA)	• Speaker: Paul Kallukaran, Executive Director, Global Information Sciences and Analytics: Commercial
Bio IT World Conference & EXPO 21-23 April 2015 (Boston, USA)	• Workshop: Biologics, Bioassay, and Biospecimen Registration Systems: ○ Speaker: Beth Basham, IT Director, Client Services, Biologics & Vaccines Discovery (Talk title to be announced) *Pharmaceutical R&D Informatics*

- **Luncheon Presentation II: Where Science Intersects with Business – Creating Business Dashboards That Combine Data from Multiple Sources** (*Huijun Wang, Ph.D., Associate Principle Scientist, Cheminformatics, Merck & Co., Inc., Eric Gifford, Ph.D., Principal Scientist, Systems Chemical Biology, Merck & Co., Inc., Matthew Clark, Ph.D., Consultant, Life Science Services, Elsevier*)
  - In today's highly competitive pharmaceutical environment it is imperative for project teams to monitor both business movements, and scientific developments that can affect the business proposition for the program. Elsevier is collaborating with Merck to develop a series of dashboards that can bring in information from multiple sources to create views with facets for drug, target, and disease related information. These dashboards will monitor scientific information gleaned from journals, patents & grant applications to provide a rich context for monitoring project status and competitive position.
- **Panel discussion: Growing a Data Science Team** (*Moderator: Martin Leach, Ph.D., Vice President, Global Data Office, Biogen; Panelists: Johnson, Ph.D., Associate Vice President, Scientific Informatics, Merck (among other panelists from other pharmaceutical companies)*)
  - Enabling Innovative Data-driven Approaches at the Intersection of Science, Medicine & Economics
  - Assembly, Creation and Implementation of Data Science Groups for Pharma
  - The Data Scientist -- an Essential Component of Big Data Analytics – Difficult to Identify
  - What are Data Sciences, Informatics and Bioinformatics?
  - Should data scientists be centralized or embedded within other product/functional teams?
  - How strong of a coder/programmer should members of a data science team be?
  - How much domain knowledge does a data scientist need to have?
- **Presentation: The Construction of a Scientific Modeling Culture and Technology Platform at Merck** (*Chris L. Waller, Ph.D., Director and Head, Scientific Modeling Platforms, Merck Research Laboratories*)
  - Merck Research Laboratories is undergoing a transformation in the way that it prosecutes R&D programs. Through the adoption of a "model-driven" culture, enhanced R&D productivity is anticipated. To support this

	emerging culture, an ambitious IT program has been initiated to implement a harmonized platform to facilitate cross-domain workflows and decision-making through agile persona driven data and predictive model access.

Real World Evidence & Data Partnerships Summit 14-15 October (Bethesda, USA)	• **Panel Discussion: Real World Evidence & The Digital Healthcare Space: The Next Frontier?** *(Panelist among other representatives from GSK and Open mHealth: Patirck Howiem Leaderm Customer Data and Applications and General Manager, Comsort)*
	   o As digital changes healthcare, has pharma caught on? Can mobile health revolutionize health outcomes research? This talk is a "Look into the future of RWE":
	      ▪ Are technologies like wearable devices the future sources of real world patient data?
	      ▪ Do data from wearables belong in the medical record?
	      ▪ What is the impact going to be for drug development?
	   o We'll explore the opportunities and hazards for pharma to engage in the burgeoning ecosystem of health technology services and solutions.

Appendix 4: Conceptual Architecture of Big Data Analytics

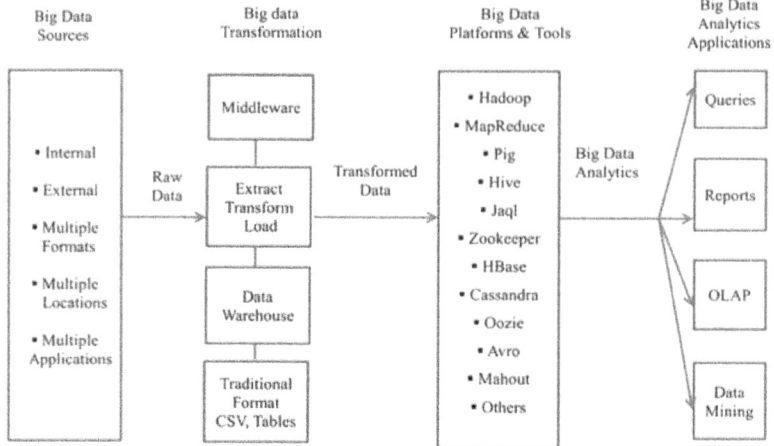

Source: Raghupathi and Raghupathi (2014), p.5

1. Healthcare data can come from several sources:
   - Internal sources such as electronic health records, clinical decision support systems, CPOE, etc. and
   - External sources, e.g. government sources, laboratories, pharmacies, insurance companies & HMOs, etc.,
   - Often in multiple formats (flat files, csv, relational tables, ASCII/text, etc.) and
   - Residing at multiple locations (geographic as well as in different healthcare providers' sites)
   - In numerous legacy and other applications (transaction processing applications, databases, etc.).

2. The raw data has to be processed or transformed:
   - Middleware: A service-oriented architectural approach combined with web services. The data stays raw and services are used to call, retrieve and process the data.
   - Data warehousing: data from various sources is aggregated and made ready for processing, although the data is not available in real-time.
   - Extract, transform, and load (ETL): data from diverse sources is cleansed

and readied.

3. Depending on whether the data is structured or unstructured, several data formats can be input to the big data analytics platform. In this next component, several decisions are made regarding the data input approach, distributed design, tool selection and analytics models (see appendix 5).

4. There are four typical applications of big data analytics in healthcare: queries, reports, OLAP (online analytical processing), and data mining. Moreover, a wide variety of techniques and technologies have been developed and adapted to aggregate, manipulate, analyze, and visualize big data in healthcare.[95]

---

[95] Raghupathi and Raghupathi (2014), p.5-6

Appendix 5: Platforms & Tools for Big Data Analytics in Healthcare

Numerous vendors—including AWS, Cloudera, Hortonworks, and MapR Technologies—distribute open-source Hadoop platforms. Many proprietary options are also available, such as IBM's BigInsights. Further, many of these platforms are cloud versions, making them widely available.

Platform/Tool	Description
The Hadoop Distributed File System (HDFS)	HDFS enables the underlying storage for the Hadoop cluster. It divides the data into smaller parts and distributes it across the various servers/nodes.
MapReduce	MapReduce provides the interface for the distribution of sub-tasks and the gathering of outputs. When tasks are executed, MapReduce tracks the processing of each server/node.
PIG and PIG Latin	Pig programming language is configured to assimilate all types of data (structured/unstructured, etc.). It is comprised of two key modules: the language itself, called PigLatin, and the runtime version in which the PigLatin code is executed.
Hive	Hive is a runtime Hadoop support architecture that leverages Structure Query Language (SQL) with the Hadoop platform. It permits SQL programmers to develop Hive Query Language (HQL) statements akin to typical SQL statements.
Jaql	Jaql is a functional, declarative query language designed to process large data sets. To facilitate parallel processing, Jaql converts "'high-level' queries into 'low-level' queries" consisting of MapReduce tasks.
Zookeeper	Zookeeper allows a centralized infrastructure with various services, providing synchronization across a cluster of servers. Big data analytics applications utilize these services to coordinate parallel processing across big clusters.
HBase	HBase is a column-oriented database management system that sits on top of HDFS. It uses a non-SQL approach.

Cassandra	Cassandra is also a distributed database system. It is designated as a top-level project modelled to handle big data distributed across many utility servers. It also provides reliable service with no particular point of failure and it is a NoSQL system. A NoSQL (referring to non-relational) database provides a mechanism for storage and retrieval of data that is modelled in means other than the tabular relations used in relational database.
Oozie	Oozie, an open source project, streamlines the workflow and coordination among the tasks.
Lucene	The Lucene project is used widely for text analytics/searches and has been incorporated into several open source projects. Its scope includes full text indexing and library search for use within a Java application.
Avro	Avro facilitates data serialization services. Versioning and version control are additional useful features.
Mahout	Mahout is yet another Apache project whose goal is to generate free applications of distributed and scalable machine learning algorithms that support big data analytics on the Hadoop platform.

Source: Raghupathi and Raghupathi (2014), p. 6

SCHRIFTENREIHE MASTERSTUDIENGANG CONSUMER HEALTH CARE

herausgegeben von Prof. Dr. Marion Schaefer

ISSN 1869-6627

1   *Lena Harmann*
    Patienteninformation und Shared Decision Making im Lichte des
    Publikumswerbeverbotes für verschreibungspflichtige Arzneimittel
    ISBN 978-3-8382-0056-9

2   *Janna K. Schweim*
    Untersuchungen zum Arzneimittelversandhandel aus Verbrauchersicht
    ISBN 978-3-8382-0071-2

3   *Ansgar Muhle*
    Deutsche Gesundheitsportale im Netz
    Kritische Einschätzung anhand der gängigen Qualitätssiegel
    ISBN 978-3-8382-0086-6

4   *Elizabeth Storz*
    Psychopharmakamarkt in Deutschland
    Eine Untersuchung zu den Strukturveränderungen
    durch das Arzneiversorgungs-Wirtschaftlichkeitsgesetz (AVWG)
    ISBN 978-3-8382-0109-2

5   *Ursula Sellerberg*
    Heilpflanzen-Datenbanken im Internet
    Eine kritische Untersuchung anhand verbraucherrelevanter Kriterien
    ISBN 978-3-8382-0092-7

6   *Rüdiger Kolbeck*
    Arzneimittelfälschungen auf globaler und nationaler Ebene
    Eine Studie über das Problembewusstsein bei Patienten und Experten
    ISBN 978-3-8382-0155-9

7   *Silke Lauterbach*
    Das diabetische Fußsyndrom
    Ein Ratgeber zur Identifizierung von Risikopatienten in der Apotheke
    ISBN 978-3-8382-0182-5

8   *Judith Rommerskirchen*
    Die Arzneimittelrabattverträge der gesetzlichen Krankenversicherungen
    Eine Studie über Probleme bei ihrer Umsetzung an der Schnittstelle von Arzt und Apotheker
    ISBN 978-3-8382-0253-2

9   *Verena Purrucker*
    Möglichkeiten und Grenzen von Franchisesystemen in der zahnärztlichen
    Versorgung in Deutschland
    ISBN 978-3-8382-0186-3

10 *Stefan Prüller*
    Risiken und Nebenwirkungen auf der Spur
    Konsumentenberichte über unerwünschte Arzneimittelwirkungen als Chance für
    Krankenkassen
    ISBN 978-3-8382-0318-8

11 *Denny Lorenz*
    Development of a Standard Report for Signal Verification on Public Adverse
    Event Databases
    ISBN 978-3-8382-0432-1

12 *Kerstin Bendig*
    Risikomanagement in der Arzneimittelsicherheit
    Ansätze zur Effektivitätsbewertung von Risikominimierungsmaßnahmen in den USA und
    Europa im Vergleich
    ISBN 978-3-8382-0438-3

13 *Dirk Klintworth*
    Reporting Guidelines und ihre Bedeutung für die Präventions- und
    Gesundheitsförderungsforschung
    ISBN 978-3-8382-0448-2

14 *Judith Weigel*
    Schwangerschaft bei Frauen mit und ohne Autoimmunerkrankungen
    Ein Vergleich hinsichtlich der mütterlichen Charakteristika und des Ausgangs der
    Schwangerschaft
    ISBN 978-3-8382-0468-0

15 *Christopher Funk*
    Mobile Softwareanwendungen (Apps) im Gesundheitsbereich
    Entwicklung, Marktbetrachtung und Endverbrauchermeinung
    ISBN 978-3-8382-0493-2

16 *Carmen Flecks*
    Auf der Suche nach Psychotherapie
    Bedarfsplanung für die Psychotherapie unter besonderer Berücksichtigung des
    Versorgungsstrukturgesetzes 2012 (GKV-VStG)
    ISBN 978-3-8382-0498-7

17 *Beate Kern*
    Arzneimittel für seltene Erkrankungen:
    Evidenzlevel der Wirksamkeitsstudien, Frühe Nutzenbewertung und Preisentwicklung in
    Deutschland
    ISBN 978-3-8382-0762-9

18 *Heike Dally*
Anforderungen an das Design klinischer Studien in der Onkologie
nach Einführung der frühen Nutzenbewertung
ISBN 978-3-8382-0933-3

19 *Malena Johannes*
Big Data for Big Pharma
An Accelerator for The Research and Development Engine?
ISBN 978-3-8382-0942-5

Sie haben die Wahl:

Bestellen Sie die *Schriftenreihe Masterstudiengang Consumer Health Care* **einzeln** oder im **Abonnement**

per E-Mail: vertrieb@ibidem-verlag.de | per Fax (0511/262 2201)
als Brief (***ibidem**-Verlag* | Leuschnerstr. 40 | 30457 Hannover)

Bestellformular

☐ Ich abonniere die *Schriftenreihe Masterstudiengang Consumer Health Care* ab Band # ____

☐ Ich bestelle die folgenden Bände der *Schriftenreihe Masterstudiengang Consumer Health Care*
____; ____; ____; ____; ____; ____; ____; ____; ____

Lieferanschrift:

Vorname, Name ....

Anschrift ....

E-Mail... | Tel.: ....

Datum .... | Unterschrift ....

Ihre Abonnement-Vorteile im Überblick:

- Sie erhalten jedes Buch der Schriftenreihe pünktlich zum Erscheinungstermin – immer aktuell, ohne weitere Bestellung durch Sie.
- Das Abonnement ist jederzeit kündbar.
- Die Lieferung ist innerhalb Deutschlands versandkostenfrei.
- Bei Nichtgefallen können Sie jedes Buch innerhalb von 14 Tagen an uns zurücksenden.

ibidem-Verlag

Melchiorstr. 15

D-70439 Stuttgart

info@ibidem-verlag.de

www.ibidem-verlag.de
www.ibidem.eu
www.edition-noema.de
www.autorenbetreuung.de

Made in the USA
Monee, IL
03 May 2026

49438570R00075